Core Surgery Interview

Edited by

Alexander Logan MBChB MSc MRCS PGCME

Andrew Fischer MBChB MSc MRCS PGCME

© 2015 MD+ Publishing

www.coresurgeryinterview.com

Published by: MD+ Publishing

Cover Design: Alexander Logan

ISBN-10: 0993113834

ISBN-13: 978-0993113833

Printed in the United Kingdom

CONTENTS

Chapter 3: Clinical

Chapter 4: Management

MORE ONLINE

www.coresurgeryinterview.com

 Access Over 250 More Interview Questions

Head over to the Core Surgery Interview website for the latest news on this year's interviews together with our online core surgery interview questions bank featuring over 250 unique, interactive CST interview questions with comprehensive answers.

Created by high scoring, successful trainees the website and question bank can be accessed from your home computer, laptop or mobile device making your preparation as easy and convenient as possible.

Contributors

Many thanks to the following surgical trainees and consultants who contributed to the text:

Langhit Kurar MBChB BSc (Hons)
Western Sussex Hospitals Trust, KSS Deanery

Ana-Catarina Pinho-Gomes MSc MRCS
University Hospital of South Manchester, Northern Deanery

Patrizia Capozzi MBChB FRCS
University Hospital of South Manchester, Northern Deanery

Yee Kuan Foo MBChB
Northern General Hospital, Yorkshire and Humber Deanery

Ammar Allouni MB.Bch MSc MRCS
Northern General Hospital, Yorkshire and Humber Deanery

Katherine James MBChB BSc (Hons)
Kingston Hospital, London Deanery

Robbie Stewart MbBch BAO Bsc (Hons)
Antrim Area Hospital, NIMDTA

Kyle McDonald FRCS (Orth)
Royal Victoria Hospital, NIMDTA

Chad Chang MBChB MRCS
Leeds General Infirmary, Yorkshire and Humber Deanery

Syed Awais Bokhari MBBS MRCS BSc
Hull Royal Infirmary, Yorkshire and Humber Deanery

Kirsty Smith BSc MBChB MRCS
Pinderfields General Hospital, Yorkshire and Humber Deanery

Sri Mahalingam MBBS Bsc MSc DOHNS MRCS (ENT)
Pinderfields General Hospital, Yorkshire and Humber Deanery

Zakk Borton BMBS BMedSci (Hons)
Hampshire Hospitals NHS Foundation Trust, Wessex Deanery

Bashar Zeidan MD MRCS PhD
Hampshire Hospitals NHS Foundation Trust, Wessex Deanery

Andrew Chetwood BMedSci (Hons) MBChB (Hons) FRCS (Urol)
Ashford and St. Peters NHS Foundation Trust

Gianluca Gonzi MD
Musgrove Park Hospital, Severn Deanery

Stephanie Buchan BMSc (Hons) MChB MRCS
Musgrove Park Hospital, Severn Deanery

Oliver Adebayo MBBS BSc MRCS
London Deanery South East Thames University Hospital Lewisham

Amit Patel MBBS BSc MRCS
London Deanery South East Thames University Hospital Lewisham

Patricia Almela MBBS
Princess Alexandra Hospital, East of England Deanery

Paul Erdman MBBS
Princess Alexandra Hospital, East of England Deanery

Lucy Maling MBChB
Royal Cornwall Hospital, Health Education South West

Michael Akinfala MBBS BSc
Guy's and St Thomas' Hospital, London Deanery

Lucy Walker MBBS MSc
Royal Victoria Infirmary Northern Deanery

Preface

Applying to core surgical training is a competitive process with around 1400 applicants competing for just under 600 training posts each year. Competition ratios in the more popular deaneries such as London and Severn are in excess of 3:1 meaning that it is vitally important to understand both the application and interview process in order to achieve the highest ranking possible and secure your job preference.

Specialty interviews in medicine today are more similar to OSCEs than traditional job interviews with candidates required to rotate through a series of interview stations each testing components of the desirable criteria outlined in the national person specification.

Written by high-scoring candidates at previous core surgery interviews this book has been specifically designed for doctors applying to core surgical training with a heavy focus on practice questions that are commonly asked at CST interviews.

Following a short introductory chapter covering an overview of the application process (we hope you already are aware of this!) and interview basics such as CV preparation and interview technique the remaining three chapters feature over 500 individual interview questions covering the portfolio, clinical and management interview stations.

Improving your interview skills is best done through practice and this book can be used in pairs or groups to practise interview questions. If you prefer to prepare alone the clinical summaries, portfolio exercises and management explanations provide realistic insight into what is expected at core surgery interviews.

For even more questions, an online question bank and plenty more resources remember to visit the companion website at:

www.coresurgeryinterview.com

We hope this book helps boost your interview preparation.

Be confident and good luck.

Alex

1 THE BASICS

1.1 Core Surgery Basics

Before starting your interview preparation it is useful to have a little background information on core surgical training and how the interview process has developed to understand what interviewers are looking for in core surgery trainees.

A Brief History of Core Surgical Training

In 2005 the modernising medical careers (MMC) programme drastically changed the face of medical training in the United Kingdom. The previous pre-registration house officer (PRHO) and senior house officer (SHO) roles were transformed into the two year foundation programme and the early years specialty training CT/ST1-2.

Previously selection into core surgical training was a mixture of local and national appointments until 2010 when the core surgery national recruitment office (CSNRO) within the Health Education Kent, Surrey, Sussex (KSS) deanery was formed to oversee co-ordinated national recruitment into core surgical training.

From 2012 England, Scotland, Wales and Northern Ireland have all used this system to select applicants into core surgical training. Initially deaneries interviewed applicants locally before submitting their score for national ranking. Since 2014 all interviews are now held centrally at an interview selection centre in London.

KSS still oversees the coordinated national recruitment for core surgery and it is well worth checking their website regularly prior to the application opening and in November and prior to interviews in January for the latest information for the year in which you apply.

Each year approximately 1300 applicants apply for around 600 core surgical training posts with current competition ratios in the region of 2:1.

Competition ratios

	2012	2013	2014	2015
Applicants	2666	1296	1370	1396
Posts	703	676	625	604
Ratio	3.8	1.9	2.2	2.3

It is important to be aware that these are national competition ratios and the most popular regions and posts will themselves have much higher competition. Essentially while competition ratios may be of interest to some we would advise trying to get as high a score as possible at the interviews to ensure you not only get your chosen deanery but also the hospital and rotation that you want.

The Deaneries

There are 15 deaneries in the United Kingdom to which you can apply for core surgical training. London is divided into three deaneries and Wales and Scotland are classed as deaneries despite their geographic area being much larger than most.

You will likely have a preference of where you would like to be for the next two years based on your current circumstance together with the rotations offered by individual deaneries and your specific job preferences.

East Midlands	Scotland
East of England	South West (Severn and Peninsula)
Kent, Surrey and Sussex	Thames Valley
London —North Central & East	Wales
London — North West	Wessex
London — South	West Midlands
North East	Yorkshire and the Humber
North West	

Choosing a Rotation

While training is standardised across all deaneries individual jobs can vary significantly even within each deanery. For example some hospital posts may position the core trainee as a junior registrar with their own supervised operating lists, on call commitments and allocated clinic sessions. Other posts (even within the same deanery) may simply put the core trainee on the SHO rota with the foundation doctors and the core trainee will need to negotiate time away from the wards or on call responsibilities to attend theatre.

As a foundation doctor applying for core surgical training it can be difficult to know which of the rotations on offer at core surgery application within each deanery offer the best training opportunities. Our advice is to ask current core surgical trainees and registrars within the deanery to which you are applying. They will have the latest, inside information on which jobs are most popular and from where successful ST3 applicants have worked.

Core Surgery Overview

Core surgical training last for 24 months during which time you will progress from CT1 to CT2 to (hopefully) ST3 and you will develop basic surgical skills and knowledge that will allow you to progress to specialty training at ST3 level. Over the two years through both on-the-job experience and teaching sessions provided at deanery level you will gain a fundamental understanding of surgical principles together with more operative experience.

You will be expected to pass the MRCS Part A and B and to boost your CV with publications, presentations and surgical experience that will enable you to progress to ST3 level.

The majority of deaneries offer four 6-month posts through which you will rotate and usually comprise of a general surgical attachment and some surgical specialty attachments such as trauma and orthopaedic surgery, vascular surgery or ENT. A few deaneries continue the 4-month rotation structure that you may be familiar with from foundation training.

Some deaneries provide a fixed 24-month programme that you will be able to see upon CT1 application while others allow trainees to select their CT2 placements during the CT1 year. This means that if you are not sure which surgical specialty you wish to apply for at ST3 you have a little more time to see which you like before making a firm decision.

Themed Training

The surgical specialties through which you might rotate during your core surgery years include trauma and orthopaedics, urology, plastic surgery, ENT surgery, hepatobiliary surgery, colorectal surgery, upper GI surgery, breast surgery and maxillofacial surgery.

It may be that you already have a good idea for what type of surgical specialty you would like to specialise in and apply for at ST3 level. The core surgery programme caters to those who do by providing a limited number of 'themed' two-year core surgery programmes. These typically comprise of a 4 or 6-month general surgical attachment and 18 months of a single surgical specialty. For example a trauma and orthopaedic themed trainee may begin with a 6-month trauma and orthopaedic placement before going to a general surgical post for 6-months and then spending their entire CT2 year in a trauma and orthopaedic rotation.

Themed training greatly increases a trainee's exposure to the themed specialty and allows for more time to improve your operative numbers and demonstrates commitment to the specialty. If you are fairly certain of your future surgical career we would highly recommend selecting a themed core surgical rotation at core surgery application as these will stand you in good-stead for applying at ST3 level.

The Intercollegiate Surgical Curriculum Programme (ISCP)

Regardless of where you train, how long each rotation is or which specialties you will rotate through the core surgical training competencies that you develop will be the same. These competencies are outlined in the core surgery syllabus devised by the Intercollegiate Surgical Curriculum Programme (ISCP). The ISCP website works in a similar way to the foundation eportfolio system and allows trainees to complete work-based assessments and links in with the elogbook system to give your supervisors and trainers a way to objectively assess you and to ensure progression over the two year core surgery programme. You will continue to use this system for the remainder of your career up to your completion of training date, the bad news is that currently trainees are required to pay a yearly subscription to use the mandatory site in the region of £350.

1.2 | The CST Application Overview

Mid November - Early December	Application Window via ORIEL
December - January	Interview long listing takes place
Mid January - Mid February	All interviews take place
Mid March	All offers made
Late March	Deadline for holding offers
Mid April	Clearing

THE BASICS

The ORIEL website recruitment portal

All applications for core surgical training must be submitted through the online application forms on the ORIEL recruitment website (www.oriel.nhs.uk). Forms will not be accepted by post, e-mail or any other medium. You can register with Oriel before the applications open and key information relating to the core surgery application is summarised on the Oriel website together with the KSS deanery site.

ORIEL is designed for candidates to manage their application through a single portal and incorporates the following:

- An initial registration process, meaning applicants only need one log in for the entire recruitment year. Some parts of the completed registration will also get automatically transferred across to the application to avoid repeating information.
- After registering, each applicant will have their own profile, it is through this that an applicant will complete the core surgery application form and be informed if they are invited to interview or offered a training post.
- Booking interviews is managed through the portal.
- All available vacancies for speciality training are listed on the website.

The Application

Applicants will make a single application to their first preference deanery, with the opportunity to rank all other deaneries for consideration.

Once the application closes all candidates will have their eligibility assessed against criteria on the core surgery person specification. Each deanery will use the same application form and all applicants that pass long listing will receive an interview.

You will be required to complete your personal details, employment history and medical qualifications. You must also declare any criminal convictions. You are required to provide referees; these should ideally be your most recent supervisors. It doesn't matter if they are surgical or not, they will only be required to complete the reference proforma if/when you are appointed a core surgical post.

It is important to be aware of the specific wording of the eligibility requirements and make sure you have copies of the required documents that will be checked on the day at the interview selection centre.

Eligibility in the application is assessed against the core surgery person specification. Applications close in early December with interview invitations sent out during late December.

The Core Surgery Person Specification

While the format and location of how applicants are selected into core surgical training has drastically changed over the last ten years the underlying characteristics and desirable criteria for selection has not. The Person Specification outlines the requirements necessary for entry into core surgical training. The Person Specification is divided into two parts: Entry Criteria and Selection Criteria.

The entry criteria lists what is required to be eligible to apply for core surgery and this includes possessing a medical degree, having (or expecting to have) obtained your foundation training competencies, being in good health and being able to fluently speak english.

The selection criteria is the more important section as it is against this that applicants will be scored during the application and interview process. The selection criteria lists both 'essential' and 'desirable' criteria in certain domains together with the stage of the selection process these will be assessed and what evidence is required to score points. There are six key domains against which applicants will be scored and it is important to be aware of these together with the 'desirable' criteria for each to know how to score maximum points during the selection process and what evidence may be required.

- Qualifications
- Clinical Skills
- Academic Skills
- Personal Skills
- Probity – professional integrity
- Commitment to specialty – learning and personal development

Application Structure

After registering through ORIEL candidates will be able to add information to the application system when it opens mid-November to early December each year. The Oriel application consists of 11 sections for core surgery. Each section is marked against the person specification and it is very important that you compare your answers to this. Section 7 (Evidence) and section 8 (Supporting) are the most important sections to answer well and in sufficient detail.

The ORIEL Application Structure

11 sections need to be completed in full prior to submitting your application.

1	Personal	Contact information and personal details
2	Eligibility	Professional Registration, language skills, right to work in the UK
3	Fitness	Criminal Records and Fitness to Practice
4	References	Three references who have supervised your training during the last 2 years. One referee must be a current or most recent consultant or educational supervisor
5	Competencies	Achievement of foundation competence Evidence of primary medical qualification: MBBS or equivalent Evidence of Advanced Life Support Certificate from the Resuscitation Council UK or equivalent
6	Employment	Full employment history UK/ Overseas Any gaps in employment of longer than 4 weeks within 3 years preceding the start date of the post, must be accounted for
7	Evidence	Additional undergraduate degrees and qualifications Post-graduate degrees and qualifications Additional achievements, prizes awards and distinctions Training courses attended Career Progression. Evidence to show career progression is consistent with personal circumstances. 18 months or less experience in surgery (excluding foundation modules) is required for CST application.
8	Supporting	Clinical knowledge and expertise Research, teaching and quality improvement Presentations and publications Management and information technology Commitment to speciality Learning and personal development Achievements relevant to a career in CST Other achievements and personal skills
9	Preferences	Application directly to deanery
10	Equality	Equality and diversity monitoring form
11	Declaration	Declarations and submission

THE BASICS

Section 7: Evidence

The evidence section on the application form includes 5 areas. The first four will make up most of your score for this section. The higher your score the better your application.

Additional undergraduate degrees and qualifications	Intercalated BSc /Equivalent Other degrees BSc /BA Includes Grade
Postgraduate degrees and qualifications	Other degrees /diplomas A PhD or MD should only be listed in this section that has been awarded for defending a thesis
Additional achievements, prizes, awards and distinctions	Include specialty and qualifying distinction Indicate if awarded as an undergraduate or a postgraduate
Training courses attended	Include relevant training courses Include courses currently being undertaken ALS
Career progression	The maximum experience in surgery for application at CT1 level is 18 months in any country. This does not include experience in foundation modules.

Section 7 scoring systems

When the application is independently scored marks are awarded based on a set scoring system. If you are aware of the requirements well ahead of time you can spread your achievements across each of the scoring domains in order to score as many high marks as possible.

A few example scoring systems for the evidence section of the application are shown on the next page.

 Prepare Early and Be Honest

Remember to prepare your application well ahead of time. While scoring maximum marks in one area is good it is important that you score highly in each section to ensure a high overall application score. Whatever achievements you list in the sections 7 or 8 make sure you have evidence to support them as any fraudulent answers may be reported to the GMC.

Postgraduate degrees and qualifications example scoring

Degree /Qualification	Rank	Example scoring system
PhD or DPhil Doctor of Philosophy	Highest score	10
MD Doctor of Medicine - two year original research-based	Middle/High score	8
MPhil Master of Philosophy	Middle score	6
Single year post-graduate course (eg MSc, MA, MRes)	Middle score	5
MD Doctor of Medicine - dissertation	Lower Score	4
Post-graduate diploma (This does not include MRCP)	Lower score	3

Additional achievements example scoring

Additional achievements, prizes, awards and distinctions	Rank	Example scoring system
Awarded national prize related to medicine	Highest score	10
High achievement award for primary medical qualification (eg honours or distinction)	Middle/High score	8
More than one prize / distinction / merit related to medical course	Middle score	6
One prize / distinction / merit related to parts of medical course	Middle score	4
Scholarship / bursary / equivalent awarded during medical course	Lower Score	2

Section 8: Supporting Evidence

The supporting evidence section of the application form encompasses other areas relevant to the person specification for core surgery. This part of the application can typically ask for short answers in prose. Section 8 is divided into 8 distinct areas closely following those of the person specification.

Clinical knowledge and experience	Details of your level of experience Level of competence Training priorities
Research, teaching and quality improvement	Audits QI projects Teaching
Presentations and publications	Presentations at regional or national level Presentations at local level Publications in journals Other publications
Management and information technology	Descriptive experiences of managerial roles or working in a team Experience with information technology
Commitment to speciality	Evidence of commitment Career objectives
Learning and personal development	Setting realistic goals Demonstrating commitment
Achievements relevant to a career in CST	Examples outside of medicine of team working, problem solving or hobbies that might improve surgical skills
Other achievements and personal skills	Achievements outside of medicine

Section 8 scoring systems
As with section 7 your answers will be scored against a set marking criteria based on the perceived level of your achievements. On the next page you will find some example scoring systems for section 8.

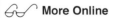 **More Online**

A full lists of the scoring systems for each section can be found on the **Core Surgery Interview** website (www.coresurgeryinterview.com). You can also find lots of free resources to help you gain maximum marks.

Clinical audit and quality improvement example scoring

Clinical Audit / Quality Improvement	Rank	Example scoring system
Designed led and implemented change through a completed audit and QI project and presented the completed results at a meeting	Highest score	10
Designed led and implemented change through a completed audit and QI project; but without presenting the results	Middle/High score	8
Actively participated in a completed audit or QI project and presented results at a meeting	Middle score	6
Actively participated in a completed audit or QI project: but with-out presenting the results	Middle score	4
Participated only in certain stages of an audit or QI project	Lower Score	2

Poster and presentation example scoring

Degree /Qualification	Rank	Example scoring system
Oral presentation at a national or international medical meeting	Highest score	6
Presented more than one poster at a national or international medical meeting	Highest score	6
Oral presentation at a regional medical meeting	Middle score	4
Shown one poster at a national or international medical meeting	Middle score	4
Shown one or more posters at a regional medical meeting	Lower Score	2
Given an oral presentation or shown one or more posters at a local medical meeting	Lower score	2

THE BASICS

1.3 The CST Interview Overview

The core surgery interviews are held at a national selection centre in London (the AMBA Charing Cross Hotel) over a week at the end of January and beginning of February.

The core surgery interview lasts 40 minutes and consists of three stations each lasting 10 minutes with time for transfer in between stations. You will rotate round all three stations but your starting station on the day will be random.

At each station you will be sat opposite two consultant interviewers who will take turns asking you questions and assessing your answers. There may also be lay-people in the interview room who will be ensuring the interviews are run in a fair manner.

The stations for the core surgical training Interview are designed to score applicants against the selection criteria listed on the Person Specification.

The stations for the Core Surgery Interview are:

- **Portfolio Station (10 mins)**
- **Clinical Station (10 mins)**
- **Management Station (10 mins)**

Each interview station is scored out of 40 based on both the content of your answers and the way in which you deliver them (communication skills).

For the clinical skills and communication skills stations you will be required to read a laminated scenario before entering the examination room. The time you take to read this scenario is included in your interview time.

Portfolio	Clinical	Management
• Interviewers have 10-minutes before the station to review your portfolio against the checklist • Candidates must complete the checklist • There are no set questions and interviewers will ask questions based on portfolio content	• 2 clinical scenarios each lasting 5 mins • The first is read outside the station • Candidates have 3 mins to read the scenario outside • The second is given 5 mins into the interview to get the candidate to think on the spot	• 1 pre-prepared 3 min presentation • 2 mins of questions about presentation • Followed by a 5 min management scenario question

THE BASICS

Portfolio station

At the portfolio station two interviewers will ask you questions about different parts of your portfolio. There are no 'set' questions as at the management and clinical stations, rather questions are asked based on the contents of the candidate's portfolio. Questions will typically follow areas of the person specification such as 'teaching', 'audit', 'leadership' etc.

As scoring is done by comparison against the person specification common questions can be prepared ahead of time. Given that interviewers will ask you questions based on your portoflio it is important that it is well-presented, key documents are easy to find and that you know the contents well. In the next section we will help you prepare your CV and portfolio and develop frameworks for structuring your portfolio answers.

 5 Common Portfolio Station Questions

These are the most common questions asked at the CST portfolio station. Chapter 2 of this book covers the portfolio station and features answers to all these questions:

1. Define the term audit
2. Tell me about an audit that you have undertaken, take me through the steps.
3. Tell me about your teaching experience
4. Tell me about a piece of research you have undertaken
5. How have you demonstrated your commitment to surgery?

PORTFOLIO STATION TOP TIPS

➕ It is very important that your portfolio folder is organised logically and clearly. Use a clear contents page at the front that outlines the topics in order. The examiners may only have 10 minutes to read your portfolio so it is important for it to be user friendly.

➕ You may also be required to direct them to specific sections when answering questions, for example they may want to see evidence of a recent audit. You will need to be able to show them exactly where this is in your portfolio.

➕ Your communication skills and interview technique together with your portfolio content will determine how well you score.

Clinical station

The clinical scenario is comprised of two, 5-minute clinical scenarios. The first is provided to you on a piece of paper before you enter the station and you will have 3-minutes to think about your answer before entering. A second scenario will be read out and/or handed to you 5-minutes into the station and you will discuss this for the remainder of the clinical station.

In the clinical scenario you will typically be asked to review a patient and make a safe clinical plan. You will need to act as though this is real life. Usually you will need to use a structured '**ABCDE**' approach and state that you would take a history and examine the patient. The examiners will then ask you specific questions. The clinical scenario is designed to assess knowledge at the level of an F2 and will not be based on a detailed surgical knowledge. Questions are commonly general surgical or orthopaedic but can come from any surgical specialty and interviewers will not know what specialties you have worked in.

Questions will test your clinical judgement under pressure (another area of the person specification) and interviewers may well ask you quick-fire questions and push the best candidates to really test their knowledge.
Interviewers simply want to know that you are safe and are able to safely and succinctly assess and identify emergent and life-threatening conditions that might affect surgical patients.

 5 Common Clinical Station Questions

These are the most common questions asked at the CST clincial station. Chapter 3 of this book covers the clinical station and features answers to all these questions:

1. Trauma call
2. Post-op DVT/PE
3. Low BP post-op
4. Loin pain *(AAA/pyelonephritis)*
5. Post-op temperature

CLINICAL STATION TOP TIPS

➕ The questions in the clinical chapter of this book cover most of the main emergent scenarios. Use an ABCDE approach to structure your answer and remember to call for senior help if required.

➕ Revise ATLS principles, read the CCrISP handbook and ensure you now the management of common surgical emergencies

Management station

In 2015 a short presentation was piloted as part of the portfolio station. In 2016 this was moved to the management station to aid timings.

Prior to the management station you will be emailed a presentation topic and aksed to prepare a 3-minute presentation without powerpoint and will then answer questions from the interviewers relating to the presentation for 2-minutes. The topic of the presentation will relate to the person specification in some way and you will be scored on your communication skills, content and timings. 3-minutes is very short for a presentation and it is important that you focus on a few salient points only and follow the advice in the communication skills and interview technique section of this chapter to score well.

The second part of the station involves talking through a 'management' scenario. Typically this is a non-clinical, problem-solving exercise that is best approached by using a set framework as suggested later on in this chapter. Many candidates find this the most challenging station as knowing how to structure and deliver an effective answer is tricky. Our best advice is to think about what you would practically do in work, keep patient safety at the forefront of any answer and involve seniors if you feel out of your depth.

---

 5 Common Management Station Questions

These are the most common questions asked at the CST management station. Chapter 4 of this book covers the clinical station and features answers to all these questions:

1. Dealing with a mistake or complication
2. Drunk colleague
3. Obstructive colleague *(s)*
4. Dealing with a complaint
5. Dealing with a difficult relative

MANAGEMENT STATION TOP TIPS

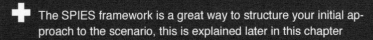

✚ The SPIES framework is a great way to structure your initial approach to the scenario, this is explained later in this chapter

✚ Keep your presentation short and on-point, questions will be a mix of typical management and portfolio-style questions as can be found in their corresponding chapters in this book

1.4 CV and Portfolio

Up until now you may have kept a fairly arbitrary CV and portfolio chronicling all of the courses you have attended and past glories as a school prefect. You probably have a vast amount of information and knowing how to present this in a manner that is both engaging and easy for interviewers to read can be tricky.

In this section we will give you the tools to help you write and layout your CV and structure your portfolio in a way that will maximise the impression you leave on interviewers and, hopefully, points scored at the structured interview portfolio station. We recommend structuring your CV and portfolio in an identical order to avoid interviewer confusion. We therefore consider both the CV and portfolio together in the below sections.

1.4.1 Layout

Knowing how to present your achievements so that interviewers spot them quickly and award you points is an art. A regular CV is usually two to three pages in length covering your previous employment, skills and extracurricular achievements. For surgeons a CV can go beyond ten pages in order to match the person specification and demonstrate achievements in all the domains necessary to be deemed an appointable candidate. The below layout is based on the authors' collective knowledge having read and reviewed over one thousand medical CVs and reviewed portfolios at interview courses.

Structure and Headings

The first step is deciding upon what headings you are going to use for your CV and portfolio. For core surgical training we recommend sticking closely to the themes described in the Person Specification to help interviewers to quickly see what you have demonstrated in each of these domains. We recommend the below headings as a good starting point:

- Personal Details
- Qualifications
- Achievements
- Appointments/Jobs
- Publications
- Presentations
- Teaching
- Management
- Research
- Audits
- Logbook
- Courses
- Extracurricular
- Statement of Intent
- References

CV Front Page

This might sound obvious but the front page is the first thing that the interviewers will see when they pick up your CV. It's kind of a big deal.
There are two real options for your front page: a cover page or straight into the first page.

Both options have advantages and disadvantages. A cover page looks neat and should feature your full name followed by qualifications to draw attention to your academic achievements. Going straight to your first page has the advantage of focussing more attention on it and reducing the amount of pages the interviewer needs to flick through. There is no right or wrong answer, just personal preference.

Cover page aside the first page should be composed of your personal details and qualifications taking up half the page. The remainder of the page should demonstrate your biggest achievements and key selling points.

The first page should be treated as the front page of a newspaper showing your most important headlines so that interviewers can immediately see what you are offering before they start looking a individual sections. This not only saves time but also gives a great first impression which is likely to stick in the interviewer's mind as he/she looks through the rest of your CV.

Ordering Your CV and Portfolio

Though your CV and portfolio should cover the domains outlined in the Person Specification (as this is what you will be scored against) there is no necessity to follow any set order for presenting these in your CV or portfolio.

We recommend putting your best areas towards the front. Interviewers have limited time to review your CV/Portfolio and will have looked through lots of others on the day. Putting your best bits first ensures that they are not skimmed through or overlooked by a tired/bored interviewer.

In practical terms if your 'teaching' section is much stronger than your 'audit' section then put 'teaching' ahead of 'audit',

Subheadings

The majority of 'main' headings can be easily divided into subheadings that make life even easier for interviewers.

For example 'presentations' can be quickly divided into 'Posters' and 'Podium' and the again into 'International', 'National', 'Regional' and 'Local'.

Chronology

When adding content under the above heading put the most recent events and work at the top with other points descending in date. This shows your most recent work easily and is the accepted format in most CVs.

THE BASICS

1.4.2 Content

Once you are happy with your layout it is time to start adding in all of your work and achievements.

Certifications First

When arranging your portfolio make sure you put your medical degree, GMC and other key certifcates at the front mirroring the 'qualifications' section of your CV.

First Page Headlines

As suggested put your best achievements on the front page under a generic heading such as 'achievements' or 'positions of responsibility', highlight your role and give a brief description (a single line) of what this entailed. These achievements can be subsequently duplicated within their corresponding section (e.g. publication, presentation etc) and provide a quick way for interviewers to immediately see your key selling points.

 Key Achievements

Book Reviewer: For Hodder-Arnold and Oxford University Press
Rota Organiser: Orthopaedic F2 and SHO Royal Hospital 2014-15
Volunteer: RCSEng School Career's Day
School Prefect: Hogwarts' School

Summary Sheets

Rather than printing out every single work-based assessment create a summary table giving an overview of the number of WBAs that you have achieved. You may also wish to include quotes from some of your 360 feedback that might help to back up your answers to questions such as 'what do your colleagues think about your communication skills?'.

How Do I Give Evidence of Audit?

Whereas publications, presentations and course attendance often come with hard copy certificates it is unlikely you will have anything official to prove that you completed an audit or quality improvement project. If this is the case use an audit summary (see box) and also print off the slides from any presentations you might have given at local departmental audit meetings.
Summaries can also be employed for research, WBAs and operations. You just need to create and print off the summary sheet and put it in the corresponding section of your portfolio.

✏️ **Using an Audit Summary**

Completed Audit Cycles:
Title: Enhanced Recovery Programme for Post-Op Patients
Location: My Royal Hospital August 2012
Role: Audit lead and identified the problem
Criteria: TKR ERP meets local guidelines
Implementing change: Education and implementation of proforma
Outcome: Average inpatient stay reduced from 5.4 to 3.5 days post op. Reducing bed costs (£225/day). Currently doing re-audit looking at patient satisfaction scores.

Should I Include...?

If this is your second or third attempt at the interviews you may well have amassed a significant volume of historic audits that you may well have forgotten about.

Keeping these in your CV/Portfolio is ok but remember that you will need to be able to discuss them in detail if you are asked about them. Removing audits from over 24 months ago is also ok but make sure you are prepared to talk about what you did in this time if you are asked.

Indeed, even if this is your first sitting including your 10M swimming certificate and Duke of Edinburgh bronze award is unlikely to score you any points but will certainly take up space. Be ruthless and try to cut our anything that won't score you points.

Verbosity

Try not to put in too much text. This takes up space and it is unlikely to be read in its entirety by interviewers with limited time. Try to explain any things such as teaching events with focused bullet points outlining what you did and what you gained.

1.4.3 Design

Finally once you are happy with both your layout and content it is time to present your CV and portfolio in a way that will make the interviewers' life as easy as possible to find key information.

Font

Size 18 Comic Sans is not going to give a good impression. Arial is simple and sized at 10 or 11 will give you a good economy of words per page. Other options are Helvetica or Times New Roman. Again there is no right or wrong option (other than comic sans) so try a few different variations to see which suits you best. Whatever you choose stick to this font for the entire CV and don't mix and match.

Colours

Colours are not required but can help draw attention to areas of your CV. In a similar vein to 'Font' try to keep things simple and, if you are going to use a colour, try to stick to one only and use it to help divide sections or to offset the header/footer area.

Dividers

A simple line can help to split up sections and divide your CV preventing it from becoming a giant block of text. Again there are a few options involving colours or boxes so try a few and decide which you like, but remember, keep it simple. Within your portfolio numbered or coloured split dividers should be used to break up sections and make it easy for interviewers to quickly flick to different sections.

Headers/Footers

The header/footer area should feature your name on each page (in case the interviewers forget). Don't go overboard and grey scaling the text can prevent it from drawing attention away from your content.

Highlight Your Name

For publications, presentations or any section where there are multiple authors make sure you highlight your name in bold text to make it stand out allowing interviewers to quickly spot your role.

Review, Edit, Review

Once you are near happy review your CV and portfolio and check for spelling errors. Get someone else to do the same and edit it again after a short break. Try to get your CV and portfolio sorted by Christmas so that you can concentrate on practising your interview technique.

Being 'good' at interviews is a skill and as with all skills it will get better with understanding how to improve and then practising. Studies have shown that impressing interviewers and scoring highly at interviews is as much about how you communicate and convey your answer as much as it is about the content of the answer itself.

1.4.4 Example CV Layout and Headings

PERSONAL DETAILS

Date Of Birth:

Address:
Telephone:
Email:
GMC Registration:

EDUCATION & QUALIFICATIONS

Postgraduate Qualifications

Medical Qualification

School Qualifications

ACHIEVEMENTS/POSITIONS OF RESPONSIBILITY

PRIZES/AWARD

END OF PAGE 1

APPOINTMENTS

Foundation Year 1

Foundation Year 2

AWARDS, SCHOLARSHIPS & PRIZES

PRESENTATIONS

International

National

Regional

Local

PUBLICATIONS

Peer-Reviewed

Abstracts

Books and Book Chapters

Non peer-reviewed

TEACHING

Postgraduate Degrees

Courses

National

Local

MANAGEMENT

AUDITS AND RESEARCH

COURSES ATTENDED

Certifications

Other Courses

MEMBERSHIPS

ELECTIVE & VACATION PLACEMENTS

EXTRACURRICULAR ACHIEVEMENTS

LOGBOOK SUMMARY

CAREER AIMS

REFERENCES

 More Online: www.coresurgeryinterview.com

- A downloadable CV template can be found on the website
- Even more articles covering CV and portfolio preparation are regularly added to the blog and newsletter

1.5 | Interview Technique

Making an impression and scoring highly at the interview stations is as much about your overall interview technique as it is about the content of your answers. Coming across as confident and a 'good' candidate is a skill and can be improved with practise. Try to utilise the below interview techniques when practising your answers.

1.5.1 | Interview Communication Skills

Interviews are not just about facts and it is important that you are aware of other factors that will contribute to your interview score and the overall impression that you leave the interviewers with.

Body language (Non-Verbal Communication Skills)

Body language is extremely important and plays a pivotal role in effective communication. It can be difficult to know how to sit, who to look at or what to do with your arms during an interview.

Sitting
A number of studies have identified the position of sitting slightly forward feet planted on the ground with hands crossed or fingers locked and forearms resting on your thighs as being the optimum position for interviews. This position makes you look calm and ready and is in between leaning over the table and slouching back in your chair. This position can be maintained for the majority of the interview and allows you to sit back slightly between questions or at the end of the interview.

Smile
Smiling has been shown to increase attractiveness by a factor of ten and will also convey confidence and personality to the interviewers. While you may be extremely nervous make sure you smile when you greet the panel and try to show enthusiasm when talking about why you want to study medicine or something that you are passionate about.

Eye Contact
Ensure that you make eye contact with the interviewers from the start. If you find holding eye contact difficult practice focussing on peoples' eyebrows when you talk to them (the eye of the other person cannot discriminate whether you are looking at their eye or eyebrow due to proximity). When listening to questions concentrate on the interviewer asking the questions, nodding to show understanding. When giving your answers make sure you make eye contact with all the panel and not just the interviewer asking the question. At least one of the interviewers will be making notes or scoring you so do not be phased if they do not maintain eye contact.

Hands

From the initial handshake to using hand gestures to enforce points your hands can help to demonstrate confidence and conviction if used correctly. Upon entering the room respond to handshakes if offered and look the interviewers in the eyes. Keep your hands on your knees or lap when listening to questions and raise them when making a firm point.

Appearance

For male applicants: smart shoes, smart suit, plain shirt and plain tie. For women a smart skirt or trousers and a shirt with or without a suit jacket will be fine. It is important that you appear smart and dress as a registrar would when seeing patients in a clinic.

Active Listening

When being asked questions sit attentively. Movements such as tilting your head or nodding in understanding demonstrate active listening and will make you appear more engaging to the interviewers.

Verbal Communication Skills

Once you have mastered body language it is time to analyse how you deliver your responses to the interviewers. An excellent answer delivered in a quiet, stuttering manner will score less than one given with gusto.

Vocal Clarity

Project your voice beyond the interviewers, sit upright and speak clearly. You will be nervous initially and may hear your voice waiver. This is entirely normal and you will settle in to things after you begin speaking.

Length of Response

Stopping yourself from talking when nervous can be extremely difficult, however, interviewers are likely to lose concentration after around 3 minutes of listening to you talk. Most structured points can be given within 2-3 minutes leaving time for further questions.

Speed

Some people talk quickly others talk slowly. Try to find a balance and don't be afraid to pause to consider the question before jumping into your answer.

Vocal Tonality

Changing your inflection and emphasising words prevents interviewers from getting bored. Think about how quickly you lose interest when speaking to someone talking about something in a monotonous, single tone voice and then think about someone who changes their tone and emphasises words. Less easy to fall asleep, right?

Enthusiasm

Following on from tonality and word emphasis make sure that you are enthusiastic when delivering your answers. Smiling and tonality make up a large portion of this and the rest is about overcoming nerves and remembering that you should be excited about surgery and the things that you have done.

Positive Answers

When answering structured, portfolio questions be sure to turn everything into a positive even when asked about weaknesses or receiving criticism. Similarly try to avoid using phrases like 'I think' or 'Maybe I would' when asked about your management in the clinical station. Be positive and use confident phrases such as 'I would manage this patient by...'. Take a look at the list of action words at the end of this chapter for more examples of how to verbally demonstrate confidence.

Presentation Skills

The 3-minute presentation given as part of the management station can seem daunting but should just be seen as an extension of the traditional interview format and an opportunity to talk, uninterrupted for 3-minutes and eat into the 10-minute station time. All of the above verbal communication skills should be utilised with particular focus on eye contact, vocal tonality and speed and timings.

Keep your content to 2-3 main points and try to show some personality in both content and delivery as interviewers will get bored after hearing the same presentation given by every candidate. Make sure you practise well ahead of time and get feedback from colleagues and keep to time.

 Vocal Tonality Practice

The sentence 'I want to be a surgeon' can be interpreted in a number of ways depending on the tonality of the delivery. For instance a person increasing their inflection towards the end of the sentence suggests a question: 'I want to be a surgeon?'. While delivery with a firm tone suggests more of a statement: 'I want to be a surgeon!'. More over emphasis of words can dramatically alter the sentence structure; 'I WANT to be a surgeon', 'I want to BE A SURGEON'.

TOP TIPS

➕ **Confidence:** Smile, make eye contact, project your voice and use positive language to convey confidence when answering questions.

➕ **Keep To The Point:** Keep your answers short and make sure you directly answer the question posed.

1.5.2 | Interview Frameworks

Although you cannot predict and prepare for every question that might be asked at interview it is helpful to have a framework to answer specific portfolio-type questions. Roughly speaking questions asked at any type of interview can be categorised into motivational, situational, opinion and specific. Having a framework will help you to logically structure your answers for both basic and more challenging questions and help you think under pressure.

Different question types will require different frameworks. Question types fall into categories or domains based on what the interviewers are testing. Whichever framework you use you should be able to cut your answer down to 3-4 solid, personal experiences and reflect on each. Remember these frameworks are guides only and it is fine to use a different way to structure your answer or only use part of the framework. You can find examples of these frameworks in action in the portfolio chapter.

Motivational and Experiential: CAMP

e.g. Why surgery? Tell me About Your Work Experience

Clinical
Academic
Management
Personal

Problem-Solving Questions: SPIES

e.g. How would you deal with this problem?

Situation
Problem
Initiative
Escalate
Support

Situational and Skills Questions: STAR

e.g. How have you shown leadership? Have you been part of a team?

Situation
Task
Action
Result

1.5.3 Interview Circuit Technique

It is important to remember that you will be rotating around an interview circuit with other candidates behind and ahead of you. Your starting station will be random and there is no 'good' or 'bad' first station. If you think an interview station has not gone as well as you had hoped don't dwell on it as you will be going directly into a new station afterwards. Below are some further tips specific for the OSCE-style of interview.

Don't Forget to...

Read The Question: Ensure you read or listen to each question and understand what the interviewers want from your answer.

Keep to Time: Make sure your answers are succinct and focussed. Time is limited as you will be moving stations and there will be little time to waffle on.

Remain Calm: If a station goes badly forget about it, don't panic and give the next station your best shot.

Be Confident: If you follow the advice in this book and practise the questions contained within together with those on the website (www.coresurgeryinterview. com) you will be well-prepared. By the time the interviews come round there will be nothing more you can do and you should feel confident and focus on your interview technique.

Content of Answers

Regardless of the interview type, interviewers will want to know about your experience, your extracurricular activities, how you deal with pressure, how you resolve problems and whether you can demonstrate empathy.

Be Personal and Specific: Talking about generic things like 'I saw a patient having blood taken' or 'I have leadership skills' will not score you as many points as using personal experiences and reflecting on what you learned.

Structure Your Answers: Structuring your answers into 3-4 headlines will make it easy for interviewers to follow and prevent you from wasting time with waffle.

Common Questions: Write out example answers for common questions and then practise them. Try not to be too scripted rather work on your delivery and enthusiasm once you are happy with your content.

Use Your CV As A Guide: Interviewers may have missed key parts of your CV or portfolio. Make sure that you talk about all the best points that you have written down and do not assume that the interviewers have read it. Your CV should be structured to say why you want to do core surgery, what work experience you have done and what you know about surgical training.

THE BASICS

Show Your Working: For tough ethical or decision-making questions be sure to talk through what you are thinking. There is often no right or wrong answer rather the interviewers want to see you logically discussing both sides of the argument or problem.

Be Positive and Sell, Sell, Sell: Interviewers want to hear how great you are and it is important that you are not bashful or reserved when telling them about your achievements and why they should choose you. Turn everything into a positive and don't undersell yourself.

Don't Give An Overview: Outlining how you are going to answer a question or explaining your framework is unnecessary and risky. One particularly awkward moment occurred when an interview candidate confidently stated there were three reasons he wanted to be a surgeon only for him to be unable to recall the third!

Read The Instructions: The communication and clinical stations will provide you with written information upon entering the station. Remain calm and read the instructions or scenario carefully. Try to mentally highlight the important points and understand what they want you to do.

Answer The Question: This might seem silly but it is amazing how often candidates do not give a direct answer or go off-topic. Make sure you understand what has been asked and avoid giving a long-winded introduction.

Other Factors

The thought of the interview can be scary and there are some other variables that you will need to consider such as how you are going to get to the venue and what happens when you get there. You will be sent detailed information regarding the interview process and venue in good time. Below are some top tips for how to stay calm around the time of the interview itself.

The Night Before: You may have chosen to stay in the city before your interview or you may be travelling up on the day. Whatever you have chosen to do ensure that you have your clothes prepared, shoes shined and know where and when you need to be at the interview location. Ensure you have all the required documentation and identification required well ahead of time. Relax and get a good night's sleep the evening before, making sure you set your alarm to wake up in good time the next morning.

On the Day: Get up in good time and have a proper breakfast. Make sure you factor in traffic if you are driving to the interview location. Upon arriving at the venue you will need to register so that the organisers know that you have arrived. Occasionally your interview time slot may have been altered. If this is the case don't panic and go with the flow. There will be refreshments provided and you will be told where you can wait before the interview.

An interviewer or facilitator will usually call you in once they are ready. Upon entering greet and shake hands with the interviewers ensuring that you try to appear as confident as possible.

THE BASICS

1.5.4 What The Interviewers Say

We asked a selection of experienced interviewers to give their opinions on what makes the difference between a good candidate and an excellent candidate. Here is what they had to say:

"*The biggest challenge of any interview candidate is answering the questions posed in a way that incorporates your best points in a concise format. Your interview station time is limited. This can be especially difficult when asked a very broad, open question such as 'Why should we choose you?'*"

"*As an interviewer I can tell you that the best candidates are the ones who answer the questions posed in a logical and structured format and who have clearly thought about how they will answer the common questions.*"

"*Candidates who appear confident, with good body language and vocal intonation have often acquired this through previous interview or public speaking experiences. The more formal interview practice that you do the more relaxed you will be on the day of the real thing and this will translate into a more confident performance.*"

"*Ask any interviewer what separates the best and worst interview candidates and they are likely to respond with a single word 'waffle'. (Most) interviewers are human and will be interviewing candidates for the entire day of interviews. Think about the last time you spoke with someone, maybe a friend or relative, who told a long and boring story. It can be difficult to stay focused and retain information when candidates talk for longer than 3-4 minutes or repeat themselves. Preparing and practising questions with a set framework will help you to get across your best selling points in a concise format.*"

"*Some candidates struggle to sell themselves and feel awkward or boastful when asked why they would be a good doctor or why they should be chosen. The best way around this is to bring objectivity into the answer. For example, rather than saying 'I am a great leader' you may be more comfortable saying 'feedback from my supervisors and peers highlights my strong leadership skills'. You should of course back this up with a specific example such as when you captained a sports team or led a crash call.*"

1.5.5 CV and Interview Action Words

One way to really sell yourself in both your application and interview is to make sure you choose appropriate action words that match the corresponding skills that are being assessed.

Below is a list of action words that you may wish to use when writing your application and CV and when answering interview questions to make your answers sound more positive and assertive.

Leadership Skills

Administered
Appointed
Approved
Assigned
Attained
Authorized
Chaired
Considered
Consolidated
Contracted
Controlled
Converted
Coordinated
Decided
Delegated
Developed
Directed
Eliminated
Emphasized
Enforced
Enhanced
Established
Executed
Generated
Handled
Headed
Hired
Hosted
Improved
Incorporated
Increased
Initiated
Inspected
Instituted
Led
Merged
Motivated
Originated
Overhauled

Oversaw
Planned
Presided
Prioritized
Produced
Recommended
Reorganized
Replaced
Restored
Reviewed
Scheduled
Streamlined
Strengthened
Supervised
Terminated

Communication Skills

Addressed
Advertised
Arbitrated
Arranged
Articulated
Authored
Clarified
Collaborated
Communicated
Composed
Condensed
Conferred
Consulted
Contacted
Conveyed
Convinced
Corresponded
Debated
Defined
Described
Developed

Directed
Discussed
Drafted
Edited
Elicited
Empathised
Enlisted
Explained
Expressed
Formulated
Furnished
Incorporated
Influenced
Interacted
Interpreted
Interviewed
Involved
Joined
Lectured
Listened
Mediated
Moderated
Negotiated
Observed
Outlined
Participated
Persuaded
Presented
Promoted
Proposed
Publicized
Reconciled
Recruited
Referred
Reinforced
Reported
Resolved
Responded
Solicited
Specified

THE BASICS

Spoke
Suggested
Summarized
Synthesized
Translated

Research Skills

Analysed
Clarified
Collected
Compared
Conducted
Critiqued
Detected
Determined
Diagnosed
Evaluated
Examined
Experimented
Explored
Extracted
Formulated
Gathered
Identified
Inspected
Interpreted
Interviewed
Invented
Investigated
Located
Measured
Organized
Researched
Searched
Solved
Summarized
Surveyed
Systematized
Tested

Teaching Skills

Adapted
Advised
Clarified
Coached
Communicated
Conducted
Coordinated

Critiqued
Developed
Enabled
Encouraged
Evaluated
Explained
Facilitated
Focused
Guided
Individualized
Informed
Instilled
Instructed
Motivated
Persuaded
Set Goals
Simulated
Stimulated
Taught
Tested
Trained
Transmitted
Tutored

Helping Skills

Adapted
Advocated
Aided
Answered
Assessed
Assisted
Clarified
Coached
Collaborated
Contributed
Cooperated
Counselled
Demonstrated
Educated
Encouraged
Ensured
Expedited
Facilitated
Familiarize
Insured
Intervened
Motivated
Provided
Referred

Rehabilitated
Presented
Resolved
Simplified
Supplied
Supported
Volunteered

Organisational and Management Skills

Approved
Arranged
Catalogued
Categorized
Charted
Classified
Coded
Collected
Compiled
Corresponded
Distributed
Executed
Filed
Generated
Implemented
Incorporated
Inspected
Logged
Maintained
Monitored
Obtained
Operated
Ordered
Organized
Prepared
Processed
Provided
Purchased
Recorded
Registered
Reserved
Responded
Reviewed
Routed
Scheduled
Screened
Set Up
Submitted

2 PORTFOLIO

2.1 | Motivational Questions

2.1.1 | Why should we choose you?

Alternative Questions
- Tell me about your CV
- Tell me about yourself
- What will you bring to the specialty?

What interviewers are looking for

This is an extremely popular interview question and is designed to give you the opportunity to open up to the interviewers and tell them why you should be selected. The open nature of the question allows you to talk through your CV highlights and demonstrate your personality to the interviewers.

How to answer

Broad, open, background questions can seem daunting and are tricky to answer well. Remember the portfolio station is your time to summarise your most impressive achievements and it is important that you are enthusiastic about your accomplishments and provide your answers in a structured manner to help interviewers score you. Interviewers are not looking for a long, autobiographical journey through your CV but rather want to know your key selling points in each domain outlined by the person specification and consequently your suitability for selection into core surgery.

The **CAMP** framework of Clinical, Academic, Management and Personal is a good way to create a coherent answer. Don't stick precisely to this order, instead put your achievements with the most impact first. Alternatively you may wish to structure your answer more closely to the person specification or the order in which you have laid out your CV. Any structure is fine provided it guides interviewers and prevents you from forgetting key achievements.
Try to keep each part to 2-3 minutes as time is limited and interviewers will begin to nod-off if you talk for too long!

Approach

Begin your answer confidently with a positive statement of your greatest achievement. You do not need to state that you should be chosen over other candidates but should present the interviewers with evidence of outstanding accomplishments that follow the person specification. Whatever achievements you select be sure to reflect upon them and say why they will make you a good colleague.
The next page contains some examples of achievements you may wish to use when structuring your answer.

PORTFOLIO

Clinical	Academic
• Log book summary • Clinical competence	• Papers you have published • Postgraduate degrees awarded • Research undertaken • Teaching qualifications, courses and sessions
Management	Personal
• Involvement with quality improvement • Rota organiser • Committee member • Organising events/course • Writing books • Updating guidelines	• Personal strengths backed up by WBAs • Extracurricular achievements • Sports, musical instruments, etc.

Example

 "I am most proud of my logbook which I have cultivated in my current DGH. I can safely perform laparoscopic and open appendectomies with supervision, and have performed over ten DHS and over twelve hip hemiarthroplasties to a very high standard, in addition I am able to make correct, efficient management decisions for emergency patients while on call, and have rapidly developed my skills in elective clinics to the point that I see patients independently. I will take these skills forward and continue to develop them in my role as a core trainee"

Exercise

> ### ✎ Write It Out
>
> Write out an example answer with four paragraphs covering the **CAMP** structure. Use personal examples and link them to buzzwords and the person specification. Don't worry about it not being perfect first time, just do it and then come back and edit it so that you have a basic template for this common interview question.

TOP TIPS

➕ **Selling Yourself:** This can prove challenging as candidates do not wish to come off as overconfident or cocky. Rather use examples and feedback to demonstrate how good you are e.g. 'My 360 appraisal graded my communication skills as excellent'.

➕ **Be Positive and Sell, Sell, Sell:** Interviewers want to hear how great you are and it is important that you are not bashful or reserved when telling them about your achievements and why they should choose you. Turn everything into a positive and don't undersell yourself.

➕ **Be Personal:** Talking about generic things like 'I have leadership skills' will not score you as many points as using personal experiences for example 'I demonstrated my leadership skills managing a woman with a post-partum haemorrhage, I was the first to the scene and performed an ABC assessment followed by bimanual compression whilst directing other team members individually in the room. I learnt multiple things including...'

➕ **Mind Map:** Use a mind map or just jot down your main headings *(CAMP)* and then add in your own personal examples under each term. This will help you to remember all the things you have done and structure your answer under pressure.

PORTFOLIO

2.1.2	What is your greatest strength?

Alternative Questions
- What is your unique selling point?
- What are you most proud of?
- What makes you stand out from everyone else applying?
- What is the strongest area of your CV?
- What is your greatest personal strength?

What interviewers are looking for:

Your key selling points that make you suitable for core surgery.
To establish whether your strengths are suitable for core surgery.
To gain insight into your character and self-confidence.

How to answer

Everyone has strengths and weaknesses. To answer this question well and score maximum points it is not simply a case of reciting a list of as many strengths as possible but rather selecting a few of what you consider to be the strongest areas of your CV. Use examples from your CV to demonstrate that these strengths are proven and, most importantly, reflect on how they relate to core surgical training.

 Choose and reflect on a CV strength

Strength: Teaching
CV Example: Attaining a postgraduate certificate in teaching
Reflection: The audience preferred interactive teaching to power point teaching. Spontaneous discussions were effective, lots of individuals were keen to reflect on their experiences with patients and I developed discussions around this.

How to avoid sounding arrogant

Most medics are bad at selling themselves and are worried about sounding overconfident when asked to talk about their achievements. While it is true that appearing arrogant will likely go down poorly with interviewers under-selling your achievements is equally as detrimental.

An easy way to get around this problem is to put examples from your CV at the centre of the discussion rather than yourself.

For example a candidate who says:

'I am excellent at communicating with patients' may come across as arrogant.

Whereas a candidate who says:

'My greatest strength has been highlighted through my 360 degree feedback where my communication skills were rated as excellent by 10 separate raters'

This not only provides evidence behind the claim but also puts the comparative term 'excellent' on the communication skills.

In essence rather than saying you are excellent it is your communication skills that are excellent and others have said this not just you.

Approach

You can structure this answer using **CAMP** or using a clinical and an extra-curricular achievement.

You might also like to use an umbrella term such as 'teaching' or 'research' as your strength and then go on to elaborate about individual papers, degrees, teaching sessions etc. that you have given.

Clinical:	Extracurricular:
• Publication • Organising conference • Updating guidelines • Postgraduate degree • 360 appraisal	• Marathon • Triathlon • Team sports • Teaching yourself language/ instrument etc

Example

 "I have many things that I am proud of including writing medical text-books, completing an MSc and receiving excellent feedback from patients and peers. But the two things I consider my greatest achievements are my organisational skills and my teaching skills. I demonstrated both of these when I organised a regional teaching day for foundation doctors which required me to locate a venue, arrange speakers, set a programme for the day and teach on practical workshops. 30 foundation doctors attended the teaching day with consultants lecturing and running surgical skills workshops. This experience will prove invaluable when teaching juniors and when organising my time between gaining operative experience and improving my CV during core surgical training."

TOP TIPS

Selling: The key to this question *(as with many others)* is that even if the examples you give are fairly ordinary you need to make them sound like they are fantastic achievements that you are proud of.

Reflect: Remember that points are awarded for why the achievement is so special and how it relates to surgery. Make sure you reflect on the underlying skills and values and try to use the person specification to relate back to core surgery.

2.1.3 What is your biggest weakness?

Alternative Questions
- What can you improve?
- How can your CV be improved?
- What is the weakest area of your CV?
- 'X' is not very good on your CV. What have you done about it?

What interviewers are looking for

To see how you react when presented with a direct, negative question or statement (essentially being put under pressure).
To ascertain your insight and self-awareness for areas of improvement.
To identify areas for improvement and to understand why that area is weak.

How to answer

Talking about weaknesses is tricky. When presented with a negative question under pressure some candidates may panic or may even fall into a depression where they agree with the interviewers that an area of their CV is particularly weak and talk themselves out of a job!
The key to this question is turning your weakness into a positive and leaving the interviewers with a feeling that you have identified an area lacking in your CV and have then done something about it.

Approach

Unless asked specifically about a personal weakness always try to use an area of your CV or professional weakness that can be easily be improved. In the unlikely event that a personal weakness is asked for try not to pick anything too serious and choose something that can be easily corrected.
You can structure your answer in a similar way to 'your greatest strength' and after mentioning the weakness reflect on how it is in fact a positive.

 From Across The Table: Interviewer's Tip

Don't do as several candidates have done in the past and say 'I have no weaknesses' as you will not score highly and interviewers are likely to make your life very difficult for the remainder of the station. Also try not to inject any humour as one candidate did when he simply replied 'Kryptonite'.

PORTFOLIO

Example: CV weakness

"It is important to have insight into areas that can be improved. From my CV despite completing an MSc in surgical sciences I consider my experience of high quality research to be lacking. While being at a DGH has enabled me to gain a huge amount of operative and clinical experience there have been limited opportunities to undertake research projects. To remedy this I contacted the Professor at the major regional research department and organized a research project looking at the effects of hamster wheels on guinea pigs."

Or a personal weakness that is relatable:

"I have high standards and like efficiency I therefore get frustrated when there are delays in collecting patients and dead time between surgical cases. I highlighted this as an area for improvement and found that it is important to take a step back, let staff do their jobs and see if there are practical ways to improve efficiency. I have recently set up an audit looking at theatre staffing levels for elective cholecystectomies as this was one of the major causes in list delays."

PORTFOLIO

TOP TIPS

+ Choosing a Weakness: Don't choose anything too bad, rather select something that is relatable and can be improved.

+ Don't Dwell On It: Touch briefly on the weakness and then quickly move the interview towards more positive things.

+ Identification and Initiative: Points will be awarded for both identifying a weakness and then demonstrating that you have used your initiative and done something to remedy or improve that weakness. Examples might include finding a mentor, undertaking an audit or research project, attending a course or simply reading up on a topic.

+ Follow On Questions: Be prepared for interviewers to push you for more areas of weakness. One candidate was asked for four further examples of areas that could be improved!

2.1.4	**Why are you applying for core surgery?**

Alternative Questions
- Why do you want to be a surgeon?
- Surgical training is long. Why bother?
- Why have you applied for this post?
- What do you like most about this specialty?

What interviewers are looking for

Interviewers want to know that you fully understand what the job entails, that you have researched the entry and selection criteria and that you are enthusiastic for a career in surgery.

How to answer

This is a motivational question and is again open and broad in scope. As with all open, motivational questions you need to present a succinct, focused answer covering key points that relate to the person specification while highlighting your understanding of what the role entails.

Thus you should not only explain your own motivations for applying but also imply why you are a suitable candidate for selection.

Having done your research and having read the introductory chapter of this book you should have a basic idea of what interviewers are looking for and you should give your answer in an enthusiastic manner. Remember the interviewers are surgeons who (hopefully) enjoy their job and you should too.

Approach

Your answer may wish to utilise the **CAMP** structure or a variant such as just personal and academic. Alternatively you may also wish to use a chronological, story-based framework to guide your answer recounting when and why you first decided upon a career in surgery and what you subsequently did to make that a reality.

Whatever reasons you have for doing surgery make sure that they are personal and you are enthusiastic. The table on the next page summarises some key aspects of the specialty.

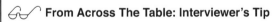 **From Across The Table: Interviewer's Tip**

Remember that it is not just what you say but also how you say it. Smile and be enthusiastic about doing surgery as a career. Interviewers will be able to spot candidates who are not convincing and it is nice for interviewers to hear how great their day job can be.

Clinical	Academic
Challenging, wide range of subspecialties Patient mix (young vs old, well vs unwell) elective and emergency procedures Able to make immediate impact to patients' lives Enjoy operating and receiving immediate feedback from trainers Be involved in prevention, treatment and follow-up of patients Interventions can rapidly and dramatically improve quality of life for patients	Evidence-based approach, strong research component, strong interface with technology, industry and MDT. Opportunity to teach practical skills and learn from peers and experienced surgeons, lifelong learning continual advances.

Management	Personal
Opportunity to improve care on a wider scale Develop organisational skills such as arranging lists, organising teaching or rotas	Personal experience of surgery Relative with illness Enjoy fast-pace Enjoy pressure Enjoy practical skills Find it fun and challenging and it helps people

Example

The below example uses a combination of the **CAMP** framework and a chronological structure to convey both motivation and suitability for selection.

 "During medical school I enjoyed my surgical placements the most out of all medical specialties. In particular I enjoyed the practical nature of surgery and the ability of surgeons to quickly diagnose and improve the health of a mixture of emergency and elective patients. I subsequently set up a surgical society for students and upon graduation selected surgical foundation rotations and researched what was required for selection and progression in surgery. I attended BSS and ATLS courses and enjoyed learning key surgical principles and pathology required to pass the MRCS Part A. My passion for both teaching and research together with my ability to work under pressure and enjoyment of technical skills make me determined to progress through core surgical training and onto higher training."

PORTFOLIO

2.1.5	What do you like least about the specialty?

Alternative Questions
- Tell me some negatives about a career in surgery?
- Is surgery always fun?
- Do all surgical trainees enjoy their jobs?

What interviewers are looking for

Interviewers want to know that you are aware of the potential negative aspects of a career in surgery. They are looking for insight and awareness so that potential difficulties do not come as a surprise to you if you are selected.

How to answer

Like the question about weaknesses this is all about making sure that you show that you have made an attempt to do something about the thing that you dislike. Choose an example that all surgical trainees might find tedious and remember to give both a personal example of your experiences of this together with some suggestions to improve or ways to deal with the problem.

 From Across The Table: Interviewer's Tip

Do not come across as too negative and try to avoid making it personal. This is not an opportunity to express your views on the decline of the NHS simply highlight a negative and move on.

Approach

You may not have been immersed in a surgical specialty to know all the minor bugbears. Think about what registrars or consultants complain about (remember medics love to complain!). Some common examples are listed below:
- The European Working Time Directive limiting training opportunities and creating shift-patterns
- The decline of the traditional surgical 'firm' due to the EWTD and training reforms with doctors more frequently rotating between jobs
- The role of management and service provision in limiting time and opportunities for training
- The length and cost of surgical training
- The loss of surgeons to Australia and increase in the number of under-filled shifts
- The focus on the 4-hour wait in emergency departments rather than patient care

PORTFOLIO

Example

 "Because I very much enjoy surgical there are certain things that I have found frustrating. Influence of industry, finance and management on patient operations and training."

The above is a good answer but you will need to expand on it and reflect if you wish to score maximum marks.

Better example with reflection

 "From my experience patient surgeries may be delayed if the correct kit has not been ordered or is not on the shelf and trainees are increasingly asked by management to provide service provision on non-teaching lists rather than be learning from experienced surgeons."

 "I think that trainees should be more involved with local management and liaising with industry/scrub staff to ensure training is maximised and kit is available. I have organised a quality improvement audit looking at delays to theatre..."

2.1.6 What are your short or long term goals?

Alternative Questions
- Where do you see yourself in 5 or 10 years time?
- What kind of surgeon would you like to be?

What interviewers are looking for

Interviewers want to know that you have a career plan and have thought about what you will be doing during your surgical training years. In years ST6-ST8 you will be focussing on a sub-specialist interest. It might be worth considering where your interests could potentially lie or an area that you are considering getting more experience in.

How to answer

This question looks at your planning and commitment to the specialty. This is an opportunity to highlight projects you may have started such as higher degrees or research and talk about how you plan on completing them. Think about what stage of surgical training you will be at. In 5 years you will be a registrar and in 10 years you will be on fellowship or will have just started as a consultant.

PORTFOLIO

Approach

Begin with short term goals and use the **CAMP** framework to structure your answer: what projects are you doing, what degrees are you doing, what operative experience are you aiming for.

Structure your long-term goals in a similar fashion. Will you be on fellowship, what kind of hospital will you be working in, what specialty will you be working in, where will you be in your personal life.

Example

 "In the next 6 months I will be completing my MSc in education and hope to have published my project on...

 In the future I would like to be a consultant specialising in minimal access surgery in a teaching hospital..."

Exercise

 Write out your career goals

Write a short summary of where you see yourself in 6-months, 1 year and 5 years time. Be specific and if you plan to sit an exam or undertake some research write these down.

2.2 | Situational Ability Questions

2.2.1 | How would you describe your communication skills?

Alternative Questions
- Are you a good communicator?
- How have your communication skills made a difference?
- How would colleagues describe your communication skills

What interviewers are looking for

Interviewers are looking for specific examples that demonstrate good communication skills. They also want to see insight into the importance of communication skills and how they can be developed.

How to answer

Communication skills can be difficult to quantify, luckily your WBAs, patient feedback and teaching feedback provide plenty of ammunition to prove how good your communication skills are.

If you have struggled with communication skills but have done something about it such as attending a course and shown improvement this is also a good example.

Approach

Rather than simply talking about your 'communication skills' try to give specific examples of communication elements such as:

- Explaining a procedure/diagnosis
- Breaking bad news
- Active listening to a patient
- Showing empathy
- Dealing with an angry relative
- Negotiating an urgent scan or investigation

Use either examples from your portfolio or short work-based examples of your communication skills in action. For the later the **STAR** framework of situation, task, action, result/reflection can be used to structure your explanation of how your communication skills led to a result and how you reflected on this.

Example

 "I believe that I have excellent communication skills as demonstrated by my 360 degree feedback and when effectively consenting patients for surgery, discussing treatment options in clinic and giving regular teaching

PORTFOLIO

sessions to large audiences. Specific examples can be shown in my portfolio such as feedback from a recent surgical career day that I organised for medical students at which I gave lectures covering the key surgical emergencies."

TOP TIPS

 Selling Yourself: This can often prove challenging as candidates do not wish to come off as overconfident or cocky. Rather use examples and feedback to demonstrate how good you are. E.g. 'My 360 appraisal graded my communication skills as excellent'

2.2.2   Is empathy important for surgical trainees?

Alternative Questions

- Give an example when you showed empathy to a patient.
- How have your communication skills influenced a patient's management?
- Tell me about a case that affected you emotionally

What interviewers want

All doctors need to possess empathy to be able to appreciate the emotions of patients that they are treating. Interviewers are looking for evidence from your work-based assessments if possible and an example of a case where you were able to empathise with a patient in a way that impacted their care in a positive way.

How to answer

You should consider this question an extension of your communication skills answer with focus specifically on building rapport and empathising with a patient. Think of a time that you have used your communication skills to help a patient or of a case where you felt particularly for a patient. This could be as simple as putting an anxious patient at ease about an operation or breaking bad news to family members in a supportive way.

From Across The Table: Interviewer's Tip

Story Telling: Use personal examples that tell the interviewers a story. This will be more engaging than listing things and will also demonstrate insight into patient care.

Approach

Select an example that demonstrates your communication skills and use the **STAR** framework reflecting on how your empathy improved things for the patient.

Example

 "A 48-year-old lady with back pain asked to speak with me as the patient and her husband were unhappy with her care during a weekend on-call period. She had a small L4/5 disc bulge but no other abnormality on MRI and was refusing to take pain relief or mobilise. I spoke with them in a quiet side room and asked a nurse to hold my bleep and inform me only if there was an emergency. I could tell from their body language and tone that they were unhappy and I used empathy and active listening to establish that they felt they did not understand what was going on. I then succinctly conveyed the diagnosis and treatment plan in an understandable way and encouraged the patient to mobilise with pain relief to facilitate her recovery. I also explained that she would be followed up by the musculoskeletal physios and could return if she developed any neurology. I know this was effective as the nursing staff noted that the family were happy with the outcome and the patient began to mobilise and was discharged the following week."

PORTFOLIO

2.2.3 | Are you a good team player?

Alternative Questions

- Give an example of your teamwork skills
- Do you work better alone or as part of a team?
- Tell me about a team you have been in
- What is teamwork?

What interviewers are looking for

Teamwork is an essential part of surgical training, whether you are in theatre with the scrub and anaesthetic team, part of a trauma call or simply on the ward with the nurses and other SHOs. Interviewers want to know that you understand the core components of being a team player and work well both alone and as part of a team.

How to answer

Your answer should convey three key facts:

- You are able to communicate and work effectively with others
- You are able to appreciate the roles and viewpoints of other team members

- You are able to make a valuable individual contribution to the team

Use specific, work-based examples that can be backed-up with evidence from your work-based assessments to highlight effective teams that you have been a part of. Remember to reflect on the experience and to focus on aspects of a good team player (see box).

Qualities of a good team player:

- Understands their role and how it fits in with the overall team.
- Is reliable, consistent, works hard, seeks help appropriately, takes initiative
- Treats others with respect
- Appreciates the role of others, approachable, responds to requests, allows others to perform their role, offer support when required
- Flexible and able to compromise
- Can adapt to changes, can consider different viewpoints, can compromise with other team members
- Communicates and listens
- Expresses thoughts clearly, proposes solutions not problems to the team, understands and listens to other views, accepts and acts on criticisms and feedback

---

Approach

The **STAR** framework may be employed to structure your answer.

Example

 "I am an excellent team player as outlined by my 360 appraisals and the results of projects such as...

Situation: Writing a paper/book
Task: I was responsible for co-authors and contributors and was required to motivate my peers while delegating work
Action: I was supportive and flexible if contributors were struggling with their workload. I listened to contributors and acted upon suggestions and improvements that they felt would help the text.
Result/Reflection: This experience impressed upon me the importance of maintaining good rapport with people and the paper has now been published."

TOP TIPS

 Teamwork: Think about what makes an effective team and how teams that you have been part of have functioned.

 Reflect: Remember to give examples and reflect on what you learned and the importance of team work in core surgery.

2.2.4	Are you a good leader?

Alternative Questions
- Tell us about your leadership experience
- What makes a good leader?
- Are you more of a leader or a manager?

PORTFOLIO

What interviewers are looking for

It is important that you can not only be a team member but can also lead a team. Interviewers are looking for examples of how you have led projects and people and the subsequent results.

How to answer

The difference between leadership and management can be tricky to define and certain aspects of each seem to overlap. Essentially leaders are concerned with using initiative to drive people towards a result that changes current practice. Managers are more focused on organising people to maintain current standards. Leaders change, managers maintain.

Leaders	*Managers*
Leaders drive a group forward to implement change. Leaders make decisions, organise and motivate team members	Managers organise a group to ensure the status-quo is maintained. Managers organise team members, ensure they meet deadlines and prioritise tasks

You will have been involved in situations that have required both leadership and management. These may be limited having come from F2 so try to interpret the question as 'How will you become a good leader' and discuss the qualities of good leaders you have worked with, examples of your own leadership and how you will develop these skills in core surgical training.

Leadership Roles:

- Creating a teaching programme
- Writing a book or book chapter with contributors
- Leading a cardiac arrest call
- Captaining a sports team
- Leading a fundraising drive
- Leading a quality improvement project

Approach

To answer this question think about people you consider to be good leaders and use personal examples to illustrate the qualities that they possess.
Use the **STAR** framework to help you structure your example answer. Ensure that you use personal examples of how you have led projects and utilise any work based assessments or feedback on your leadership skills. Remember to reflect on your experiences and mention how you will develop your leadership skills during surgical training.

Example

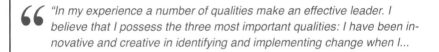 *"In my experience a number of qualities make an effective leader. I believe that I possess the three most important qualities: I have been innovative and creative in identifying and implementing change when I...*

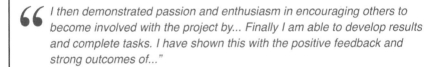 *I then demonstrated passion and enthusiasm in encouraging others to become involved with the project by... Finally I am able to develop results and complete tasks. I have shown this with the positive feedback and strong outcomes of..."*

TOP TIPS

Leadership: If you are struggling think about the best leader that you know in or out of work. What characteristics do they possess that make others listen and follow them? You may also wish to look at the action words section of The Basics chapter of this book to help you think about words and actions that imply leadership qualities.

2.2.5	Tell me about your management skills

Alternative Questions
- Are you a good manager?
- What makes a good manager?
- How do you manage people?
- Tell me about a project you have managed

What interviewers are looking for

All surgical trainees must possess management skills in order to maintain standards. Interviewers are looking for an understanding of a trainee's role as a manager, what this involves and examples of how you have demonstrated management skills.

How to answer

Managers are concerned with handling people and colleagues in order to meet set standards. Their skills are mainly organisational and are centred around analysing problems and communicating with people to maintain and achieve set goals.
Most interviewees (even at ST3 interviews) find management the most challenging area of their CV to fill. This is partly due to the ambiguous definition and partly due to perceived lack of exposure to management opportunities.

Example management roles:
- Sitting on a committee
- Organising a rota
- Quality improvement

Approach

The **STAR** framework can be used to structure your answer. Think about when you have organised and managed people or tasks.

Example

"During my trauma and orthopaedic F2 placement I was tasked with organising the SHO rota for the F2s in order to ensure it was compliant with working hours and allowed all of the team to take annual leave within the allotted time. Feedback from my supervising consultant demonstrated my strong management skills as I was able to effectively communicate with the other F2s and prioritise leave requests while analysing and organising each SHO's shifts to maintain adequate ward cover and thus patient safety. I will continue to develop my management skills during core surgical training by becoming more involved with committee roles at local and regional level to help maintain standards of surgical training."

2.2.6	Are you a good teacher?

Alternative Questions
- What makes a good teacher?
- What feedback have you had on teaching sessions given?
- Are you interested in medical education?
- What objective evidence do you have that demonstrates your teaching ability?

What interviewers are looking for

Trainees in surgery must possess a strong academic background and teaching and training future trainees has always been vital to the apprenticeship model of surgical training. Interviewers want evidence of teaching that you have been involved with together with feedback and understanding of the importance of teaching and the various methods of learning and delivering teaching.

How to answer

This open question may seem difficult to answer at first glance.

Summarise your teaching experience and use specific feedback from sessions given to demonstrate that you are a good teacher. The qualities of a good teacher can be fairly subjective depending on learning style.

The key to this question is to think of the best teacher you have had and elaborate on the qualities they possessed.

Qualities of a Good Teacher

- Enthusiastic
- Experienced
- Involves student
- Listens to student
- Understands different learning styles
- Leading a quality improvement project

Make sure you finish the question by emphasising that you possess these qualities and back the claim up with evidence from your work-based assessments. This is also a good time to talk about any teaching degrees, courses or feedback you have.

Approach

The **STAR** framework should be utilised to structure your personal example. Focus on some of the qualities that you consider good teachers to possess and make sure you try to summarise the best teaching projects that you have been involved with.

Examples of Teaching

- Undertaking a higher teaching degree
- Medical student teaching
- Departmental teaching
- Organising a teaching course
- Creating an e-learning resource

Example

 "Having completed a postgraduate certificate in medical education I could tell you many generic characteristics outlined by studies such as setting goals, creating a teaching plan, defining learning styles or respecting students however from my personal experiences the three most important characteristics are enthusiasm, being a role model and reflecting on feedback. I have demonstrated these when..."

PORTFOLIO

2.2.7 | Tell me about your best audit

Alternative Questions
- What is your experience of audit?
- What do you understand by the meaning of an audit?
- What audits have you completed?
- What quality improvement projects have you been involved with?
- How have you improved patient care in your hospital?
- What is your most recent/current audit project?

What the interviewers are looking for

Quality improvement and maintaining patient safety through regular audit are a vital part of surgery. Interviewers want to know you have completed an audit cycle and have experience of the importance of audit together with the difficulties associated with ensuring standards are maintained even after the audit cycle has completed.

How to answer

This is a chance to talk about the audit that you are most proud of.
In preparing for this question make sure you know data for all of your audits included in your application even those completed a number of years ago. Also make sure you know where the audit is in your portfolio in case the interviewers have difficulty finding it.

Audit Definition: An audit is a systematic quality improvement tool comparing current practices with set standards to maintain quality of patient care and outcomes.

Audits are part of clinical governance and are important to patients, hospitals and doctors.

- They maintain standards and outcomes in the healthcare setting.
- They help maintain patient safety.
- They help hospitals identify areas for improvement and help them meet standards.
- They train junior doctors to be analytical and improve their management skills.
- Data collected can be shared with other trusts to implement change on a larger scale.

Approach

Structure your answer by giving some background as to why the audit was important, the criteria for audit, the change implemented and the outcomes. You can use the **STAR** framework if you wish but having a structure that matches a standard audit proposal may be help show interviewers you have an understanding of the audit process.

Example

Background: "My trust had recently introduced guidelines for elective THR enhanced recovery programmes. Some of the anaesthetists had noted that there was a difference between the individual surgeons. My Consultant was keen for the department to utilise the guidelines properly. It interested me as I had little experience of enhanced recovery and it gave me the opportunity to look at current literature, which demonstrated significant improvement."

Criteria: "Elective THRs meet local guidelines using nutrition, rapid mobilisation, early catheter removal and thromboprophylaxis'.
The audit identified that catheters were often late to be removed post-operatively and the administration of LMWH was often delayed. There was also poor documentation in the surgical operation note as to a patient's suitability for enhanced recovery."

Implementing change: "Education and implementation of a proforma"

Outcome: "The average inpatient stay reduced from 3.2 to 2.1 days post THR. Reducing bed costs (£225/day). Currently doing re-audit looking at patient satisfaction scores."

TOP TIPS

✚ **Audit Summary:** It is a good idea to create a single A4 sheet summarising each of your audit projects using the subheadings above. This has two purposes; to remind you of the key points and facts of each audit and to make the audits easier to find within your portfolio.

✚ **Be Specific:** Remember to re-read all your audits. The above summary sheet will help with this but you can deflect difficult interview questions by ensuring you know specific facts such as the number of patients in a study, the timings of the study, the outcome improvement figures and where the outcomes are *(have they fallen back)* now.

2.2.8 | Tell me about your research

Alternative Questions
- Tell me about the research project you are most proud of
- What is your most recent/current research project?
- Tell me about your publications
- What research have you been involved with?

What Interviewers are looking for

Research helps to advance surgical techniques and principles and it is vital that any interventions offered to patients are evidence-based with documented, well-researched benefits, Interviewers are looking for knowledge of the importance of research, how research should be conducted, types of research and active involvement in a research project.

How to answer

This is an opportunity to be enthusiastic about your postgraduate degrees, publications and research projects. If you have little research experience or no publications talk about a current project that you are undertaking. Whatever you mention make sure you know where it is in your portfolio and all the data around it as follow up questions may catch you out.

> **Research Definition**: Research is a systematic process to answer a question aiming to create new standards of care, helping to establish best practice.

Research can be thought of as being important to patients, hospital and doctors.

Patients: Advances Surgical Techniques and Patient Care
Research advances surgery and patient care by identifying new knowledge and treatments that benefit patients.

Hospitals: Improves Hospital Reputation and Funding
Research helps units and trusts to improve their reputation and secure funding.

Doctors: Improves Knowledge of Researchers
Research helps trainees and Consultants to develop their understanding of conditions and pathologies, to back up their decisions with evidence based medicine and improves transferable skills such as analysis, problem-solving and organisation.

Approach

You should structure your answer as you would a research abstract with background, methods, results and conclusions. Alternatively if you are in the process of conducting research you may wish to describe the specific steps you have achieved thus far such as writing a funding proposal, identify a research question, setting a null hypothesis, calculating the study power or applying for ethics approval.

Example

 "I have successfully completed two research projects and am currently undertaking a third. The research I am most proud of is a study of.... published in Injury. The study looked at...and concluded that... I have also completed an MSc in... and am currently at the data collection stage for a study looking at..."

TOP TIPS

➕ **Selling Yourself:** This can often prove challenging as candidates do not wish to come off as overconfident or cocky. Rather use examples and feedback to demonstrate how good you are e.g. 'I successfully received funding for my research project'

➕ **Be Specific:** Similar to the audit section above make sure that you know all the facts and figures related to your research.

PORTFOLIO

2.2.9	Probity: Tell me about a mistake you have made

Alternative Questions
- Tell me about a time you have shown integrity
- Have you had any operative complications?
- Have you received a complaint?

What interviewers are looking for

All doctors must demonstrate probity and honesty as outlined by the GMC. Interviewers want to know that you are honest and can take responsibility for any mistakes you may have made.

How to answer

Everyone has made a mistake or had an operative complication and if you have not you will do in the future. The key aspect is that any mistake or complaint should be acknowledge, investigated and then treated as a learning point to see if current practices can be improved. Select a mistake that was not serious but has a good learning point attached. As with all 'negative' questions do not get phased but rather see this as an opportunity to turn the question into a positive. Make sure you are honest in your account and remember that the most important part is reflecting and acting on the outcome.

Approach

The **STAR** framework can be used to answer this question. Remember that interviewers may push you for more mistakes and learning points so ensure you have a few good examples prepared.

Example

"During a busy oncall period I was asked by a ward nurse to mark a patient who had been consented but not marked and was with porters waiting to go to theatre. I quickly read the notes and consent form and explained to the patient I needed to mark his arm. He put forward his left arm towards me and I went to mark the arm with the marker before quickly realising that it was actually the opposite elbow that was to be operated on. I apologised to the patient and marked the correct arm. My mistake would have delayed his surgery and could have led to a never event of wrong site surgery. Subsequently I looked up the incidence of wrong site surgery (1/10000) and now ensure that I calmly look at imaging, patients notes, consent form and ask the patient prior to marking the surgical site."

PORTFOLIO

2.2.10   Risk: Are you involved with risk management?

Alternative Questions
- How do doctors manage risk?
- When did you last perform a risk assessment?
- How are you involved in maintaining patient safety?

What interviewers are looking for

Interviewers want to see that candidates have knowledge and awareness of risk and patient safety. All doctors are involved in assessing risk and interviewers want personal examples of your involvement.

How to answer

This can seem like a fairly ambiguous question and requires some understanding of what risk management actually is. Risk management is one of the pillars of clinical governance.

Risk can be divided into: risk to patients, risk to staff and risk to organisation.

Risk to patients: is minimised by adhering to national standards and ensuring that the standards are maintained. In essence clinical audit helps to minimise patient risk and maintain patient safety.

Risk to staff: is minimised by ensuring staff are immunised and are aware of work-place risks by completing mandatory trust training for skills such as manual handling and conflict resolution.

Risk to organisation: is minimised by reducing risk to the above two and by ensuring frameworks are in place to deal with organisational issues such as filling empty rota slots with locums, securing confidential data and maintaining workplace safety.

By default you will have been to and possibly taught at a departmental induction for staff and colleagues, which minimises staff risk. You will have undertaken a clinical audit to maintain patient safety and are involved in risk management on a daily basis when assessing and prioritising patients.

Approach

The **STAR** framework can be used to answer this question. Choose a personal example and remember to reflect on what you learned relating to risk.

Example

 "I am regularly involved in risk management when assessing patients for theatre, identifying at risk, high ASA graded patients and ensuring that they are pre-operatively optimised. I am again involved in risk management when the patient reaches theatre and I take part in the WHO

surgical checklist to ensure that set criteria are met before the patient is operated upon. Finally I am regularly involved in audits and have recently undertaken an audit of VTE risk assessment for new patients admitted to the ward to ensure that standards are being maintained and patients are receiving appropriate VTE risk assessments and prophylaxis."

2.2.11	Judgement: Can you work under pressure?

Alternative Questions

- How do you cope with stress?
- Surgery is stressful. Will you cope?
- Give us an example of a stressful situation you have been in?

What the interviewers want

Interviewers want to know that you can function effectively in high-pressure environments such as trauma calls and emergencies. Interviewers want evidence of experience of working under pressure and personal strategies to both identify stress and to cope with high-pressure, stressful environments.

High Pressure Situations

- Trauma call e.g. polytrauma
- Unwell patient, e.g sepsis post-op
- On call covering multiple patients
- Acting up, your registrar is busy in theatre with the consultant and a patient has just arrived and is peritonitic
- Covering a sick colleague, low staff
- Assisting in a life-saving operation
- Dealing with an emergency such as a cardiac arrest for suspected pulmonary embolism
- Difficult/angry patient or relative

How to answer

Regardless of how the above question is asked interviewers want a personal example of a high-pressure, stressful situation that you have identified, experienced, what you did, how you coped with it and what you learned that you will take forward into core surgical training.

Coping Strategies

- Prioritising tasks
- Seeking help
- Delegating work
- Remaining calm and thinking
- Taking a step back and assessing
- Having insight into when you are stressed
- Staying healthy, taking breaks and resting

Approach

The **STAR** framework can be used to answer this question. Remember that interviewers may push you for more mistakes and learning points so ensure you have a few good examples prepared.

Example

 "I am able to identify potentially stressful situations and work under pressure to a high level as demonstrated by 360 feedback. When working on a busy medical admissions unit overnight with a team member down I was tasked with clerking in over 40 new medical admissions with just the on-call registrar. The registrar was also dealing with sick ward patients meaning that I was often left alone on the unit. I identified this as a stressful situation and prioritised the sickest patients to be triaged first while ensure that I took breaks when possible and kept hydrated. When both the registrar and myself began to get overwhelmed by the number of unwell new admissions we contacted the on call consultant who came in to help with the workload. Between the three of us we were able to safely staff the unit overnight and maintain patient safety. Looking after myself while prioritising and seeking help when required will prove an invaluable experience when dealing with surgical emergencies especially in situations where either the registrar or myself are also required to be operating in theatre'."

2.3 | Specific Questions

2.3.1 | Academic

What is an audit?

An audit is a systematic quality improvement tool comparing current practices with set standards to maintain quality of patient care and outcomes.

What is the audit cycle?

Clinical audit has a number of defined stages. Stages five and re-audit below encompass closure of the audit loop.
- Stage 1: Identify the problem or issue
- Stage 2: Define criteria & standards
- Stage 3: Data collection
- Stage 4: Compare performance with criteria and standards
- Stage 5: Implementing change
- Re-audit: Sustaining improvements

Why is audit important?

Audits are part of clinical governance and are important to patients, hospitals and doctors.
- They maintain standards and outcomes in the healthcare setting.
- They help maintain patient safety.
- They help hospitals identify areas for improvement and help them meet standards.
- They train junior doctors to be analytical and improve their management skills.
- Data collected can be shared with other trusts to implement change on a larger scale.

What problems have you encountered with audits that you have conducted?

Try to use a personal example if possible. An audit that you didn't complete would be acceptable provided you say why.

Problems:
- Local process and may not be easily transferable
- Junior doctors rotate through departments meaning sustainability is poor
- Finding solutions to the problems found can be difficult
- Suggested change may not always be popular with staff or create more work for staff
- Creates more work for busy junior doctors

Example

 "I undertook an audit into ward-based VTE thromboprophylaxis to ensure that drug charts were correctly completed. After successfully completing the audit loop we were able to improve VTE prescribing. Frustratingly 6-months later standards had dropped down to their previous level and sustainability was tricky due to the junior doctors rotating and no, one person taking a lead. We therefore assigned a role to one of the senior nursing staff to ensure levels are maintained. This in itself does create more work but does ensure that standards are maintained."

What is the difference between research and audit? Is an audit research?

Clinical audit is 'a quality improvement process that seeks to improve patient care and outcomes through systematic review of care against explicit criteria and the implementation of change'.

Research is a one-off, systematic and organised way to find answers to questions. Research does not check whether you are complying with standards, instead its aim is to create new knowledge and new standards.

In essence research helps to establish best practice while audit ensures that best practice is carried out.

What do you understand about levels of evidence in research? What level of evidence is your research project?

Oxford Centre for Evidence-Based Medicine (EBM)

I RCT/Meta-analysis
II Cohort Study
III Case-Control Study
IV Case Series
V Expert Opinion

Should research be compulsory? Who should do research?

This is a somewhat loaded question as the person specification scores you on research completed.

The question wants you to give an argument for and against. You do not need to reach a firm conclusion but rather appreciate that research is important but it is not for everybody. This is also an opportunity to talk about your own research and move the interview along.

Example

 "Research is an important part of medical practise and part of clinical governance. Not every trainee has access to research centres and many in DGHs struggle to organise good research projects. Not everyone will

want to take time out to complete a higher degree but the option is there for those who do. Personally I enjoy research and have completed 3 projects..."

Describe how you would answer a research question

If you have set up your own research project use this as a personal example and comment on the steps involved and difficulties encountered.

The basic steps are outlined below:
- Literature review,
- Find supervisor with experience,
- Null hypothesis,
- Primary aims,
- Power and sample size calculation with statistician,
- Ethics committee approval,
- Cost analysis and funding approval if necessary,
- Start recruiting patients,
- Collect data,
- Statistical analysis,
- Conclude,
- Write-up,
- Publish,
- Present.

What are validity and reliability?

Validity: is comprehensiveness – does it measure what it intends to measure?

Reliability: is the error in a measurement tool or its consistency

What are sensitivity and specificity?

Sensitivity: measures the proportion of actual positives which are correctly identified as such (e.g. the percentage of sick people who are correctly identified as having the condition)

Specificity: measures the proportion of negatives which are correctly identified as such (e.g. the percentage of healthy people who are correctly identified as not having the condition)

How do you decide if a treatment is worth implementing?

All treatments should have level one research proving that they are effective in their outcome. They should be evidence-based. Once a treatment has been proven to be effective it should undergo a cost-analysis to ensure that it is practical to offer it to patients over other treatments. In a cost-effectiveness analysis, the benefits of a treatment are expressed in non-monetary terms related to health, such as symptom-free days, heart attacks avoided, deaths avoided or

PORTFOLIO

life years gained (that is, the number of years by which the intervention extends life). Cost-effectiveness analysis assesses the cost of achieving the same benefit by different means.

What is a gold standard or criterion standard test?

In medical statistics gold standard test usually refers to a diagnostic test or benchmark that is the best available under reasonable conditions
A hypothetical ideal "gold standard" test has a sensitivity of 100% with respect to the presence of the disease (it identifies all individuals with a well defined disease process; it does not have any false-negative results) and a specificity of 100% (it does not falsely identify someone with a condition that does not have the condition; it does not have any false-positive results). In practice, there are sometimes no true "gold standard" tests.

2.3.2	Teaching

What types of teaching do you know?

1 to 1 teaching
Pros: catered to the individual student, allows gaps in knowledge to be identified and maximizes participation and interaction
Cons: time consuming, heavily relies on teacher-student rapport, can be intimidating, teaching can be too paternalistic, no learning from peers.

Small-Group teaching
Pros: encourages communication and team building, facilitates problem-based learning, teacher acts as mentor guiding group discussion before ideas are shared as small groups come together at the end, students learn from each other.
Cons: some group members can take over discussion, dependent on participation, requires a set pre-course knowledge level of topic.

Didactic Lectures
Pros: Can reach a large audience, can be interactive if pushed,
Cons: not catered to individuals, does not require participation, relies on presenter and slides

E-learning
Pros: can reach large number, allow learners to learn in their own time and promotes self-directed learning, allows distance learning
Cons: needs to be well structured and formally assessed to ensure participation, asking questions can be difficult

How would you organise a weekly SpR/SHO teaching session?

This question tests your logical thinking and also your organisational skills.

If you have previously organised a course or event make sure you mention it and reflect on the learning points.

Example

"I have previously organised a conference so I would utilise my experiences from this:

- I would first utilise feedback on the existing teaching, gain insight from my peers and also outline what I would want teaching to provide
- Involve peers who could help – someone to look after finance, someone to organise speaker practicalities such as parking expenses etc.
- I would look at a national curriculum such as ISCP or FRCS curriculum to define objectives that teaching must achieve
- I would involve a senior consultant with a passion for teaching and evidence-based medicine to oversee the course and recommend speakers
- Define a format such as lectures, SGT, journal club or practical workshops
- I would find a suitable time and location for teaching to take place to maximise attendance, this could be centrally located or rotate around local hospitals
- I would budget for refreshments and ensure I get free room and AV hire to minimise costs
- For any simulation or cadaveric materials I would involve industry and acquire appropriate sponsorship
- As not everyone will be able to attend I would also try to make materials available online and institute pre-reading materials such as journal articles or key topics
- Online sign-up
- Ensure regular contact with attendees and speakers
- Gain feedback and improve subsequent sessions"

2.3.3 | Topical surgical questions

What qualities make a good surgical registrar?

Surgical registrars play a wide variety of roles in the job such as doctor, surgeon, trainee, trainer, team member, and supervisor. Think about what is on the person specification and remember to say that you posess all these qualities.

- Management
- Communications skills
- Good clinical and technical skills
- Enthusiasm, determination, diligence
- Intelligence, common sense, logical thinking
- Insight *(particularly into their limitations)*
- Empathy

As as a core trainee and then as a registrar you will often be in a position to have to call upon your senior or consultant for advice or to come in, what sort of things would you call him/her for?

There are two principal reasons to contact your senior:

- To keep them informed about things
- To obtain advice and help

In terms of clinical cases you should involve them in:

- Any case in which you feel out of your depth
- Inform of serious and higher profile cases, eg those in which there are multidisciplinary management issues
- Referral to other centres that require

What do you understand about the Francis report?

In 2007-8 high mortality rates at Mid-Staffs Trust were highlighted for emergency admissions. This led to public enquiry lead by Robert Francis QC beginning in 2010.

The final report was published in 2013 with 290 recommendations.

The key recommendations were to legally enforce a new duty of openness, transparency and candour amongst NHS staff.

How have the introduction of major trauma centres (MTCs) affected your training?

In 2012 a network of 22 major trauma centres was launched in the United Kingdom. Previously, patients who suffered major trauma were simply taken to the nearest hospital, regardless of whether it had the skills, facilities or equipment to deal with serious injuries. This often meant patients could end up being transferred, causing delays in people receiving the right treatment.

The MTC network means ambulances take seriously injured patients directly to a specialist centre where they will be assessed immediately and treated by a full specialist trauma team.

For surgical trainees this has meant that experience of managing polytrauma and significant trauma cases will only be during rotations at MTCs. More importantly both surgical and emergency trainees become somewhat de-skilled with ATLS principles when working for long periods in district general hospitals and rely on rotations at MTCs to improve their emergency trauma skills.

How much does it cost to train a surgeon and who pays for this?

The cost of surgical training in the UK is over £400 000, a third of which is funded by the trainee.

The salary of a doctor in training is currently provided for equally between the employing NHS trust and the Postgraduate Deanery, reflecting the theoretical division between the service and training aspects of the job.

The deanery funding comes from the Multi Professional Education and Training (MPET) budget. MPET is a funding stream from the Department of Health that finances the additional costs of training in the NHS.The department of health is funded by the tax payer.

Should surgical training be shortened?

Currently training a surgeon takes around 10 years following completing of foundation training. Upon completion of core surgical training and entry into higher surgical training (ST3 onwards) trainees rotate through various subspecialties before going on fellowship and specialising in a chosen field. There has been call to sub-specialise earlier and thus shorten the cost and length of training. This is a similar argument to changes made to foundation training. The arguments for are to streamline training and reduce costs and improve specialisation. The arguments against are based around the idea that all surgeons should have generic skills and trauma skills rather than only being skilled in one field.

How would you know that you are making good progress in your training?

This question not only allows you to show insight into self-assessment but also to highlight what you have achieved thus far.

The ISCP is designed to monitor your progress by keeping track of your WBAs and logbook. There ARCP summatively assesses your progress throughout the year.

On a more personal level you create set targets with your educational supervisor and compare yourself with your peers.
You can also state that you meet the person specification and have achieved both the minimum requirements for courses and exams together with more.

Who is in charge of your training?

This question may be interpreted in a number of ways.

Interviewers are looking both for factual knowledge as to the committees who influence your training but also want you as a trainee to take responsibility for your training.

 "The Royal College together with the SAC and programme directors influence training on a national and regional level. On a local level my educational supervisor and myself are responsible for ensuring that I work hard and achieve the required WBAs and operative experience as outlined by the ISCP."

Are work-based assessments useful?

This is a controversial question and it is important that you give both sides of the argument.

The ISCP suggests that 42 WBAs should be completed by trainees each year.

Example:
Positive: With a reduction in training time experiential training is not producing sufficient exposure to maintain standards therefore evidence suggests that competency-based assessments are a viable alternative.
If used properly, at the time of the assessment trainees can reflect on what they have done.

Negatives: Time consuming, often a tick box exercise with little benefit

Do you think 7-day a week care will impact surgical training?

The UK government have set targets to provide the same level of care regardless of week day. While this is largely supported by the medical profession the manner in which they proposed the reforms suggested a lack of insight into current weekend practises. The main issues raised by the royal colleges and BMA is that in order to maintain training and comply with the EWTD more money and staff would be required to safely fill compliant rotas and ensure patient safety. From a training viewpoint provided trainees are not used as a service provision to fill extra rota gaps it may well have little impact.

PORTFOLIO

3 | CLINICAL

CLINICAL

3.1 | Post-Op: Abdominal Pain

Scenario

A 32-year-old with Crohn's disease underwent an elective subtotal colectomy with ileorectal anastomosis 3 days ago. The initial postoperative period was uneventful but the patient is now acutely deteriorating on the ward. He is febrile, tachycardic, hypotensive and complaining bitterly of abdominal pain.

What would your initial management of this patient be?

This patient is unstable and requires assessment using an ABCDE approach. Airway patency must be confirmed, though it is suggested by his being able to voice concern about his abdominal pain. 15L oxygen through a non-rebreathe mask should be administered and IV access with 2 large bore cannulae secured. He is hypotensive and tachycardic and fluid resuscitation should be commenced with a bolus of crystalloid solution and catheterised. The patient is examined to assess the extent and site of peritonism and other clinical signs. Surgical seniors should be involved early, and it would be prudent to consider liaising with HDU/ITU regarding a potential transfer.

What is your differential diagnosis?

Anastomotic leak with generalised peritonitis, septic shock, haemorrhagic shock, bowel perforation, ischaemic bowel, bowel obstruction, wound infection, hospital-acquired sepsis such as line sepsis.

What investigations would aid your diagnosis?

Bloods: including FBC, U&Es, LFTs and group and save (he is in shock during the postoperative period so it would be prudent to fully cross-match blood).
Arterial blood gas: specifically for lactate.
Blood cultures

If stable:
AXR and CXR: although pneumoperitoneum may be present in the postoperative period.
CT abdomen

What is the relevance of the patients' young age and history of IBD when considering his haemodynamic parameters?

The patient is relatively young, and should be assumed to have robust compensatory mechanisms. The fact that he is hypotensive as well as tachycardic is a later sign in young, fit individuals and should alert the clinician to potentially serious underlying pathology. Similarly, patients with longstanding IBD are usually immunosuppressed and therefore could mask signs of peritonism which renders clinical assessment somewhat challenging.

The patient continues to deteriorate despite 1.5 litres of crystalloid resuscitation (with further fluids running currently). He is becoming confused and is peritonitic. The surgical registrar is en route. What is the likely management and what can you do in the interim?

The patient remains haemodynamically unstable despite resuscitative efforts. He is pyrexial and peritonitic. Septic shock secondary to peritonitis following anastomotic leak is the most likely diagnosis. Intravenous antibiotics should be promptly commenced alongside resuscitation. He is too unstable for imaging and it is likely that emergency laparotomy is indicated. The registrar is en route, but it would be prudent to alert the emergency theatre and on-call anaesthetist about an imminent emergency case. If they are not already aware, high care (ITU/HDU) should be notified as it is likely the patient will require a higher level of care postoperatively.

The patient goes to theatre and the findings are of dehiscence of the anastomosis with faeculent peritonitis. The anastomosis is resected, the rectum oversewn and an end-stoma formed. He goes to ITU postoperatively.

After his repeat surgery, the patient has a stoma. What different bowel stomas are there and how might you distinguish between them?

A stoma is a therapeutic opening in the wall of a hollow viscus. The most common types of bowel stomas are ileostomies and colostomies. They can either be temporary or permanent.

An ileostomy is formed by bringing the ileum out onto the abdomen. They can be differentiated from colostomies as they are formed to have a 'spout', rather than flush to the skin. An end ileostomy is single barrelled, and forms the end point of the alimentary tract. A loop ileostomy is double barrelled (a proximal and distal barrel) and is used to divert gut contents away from an obstruction or resection downstream. The stoma product is usually greenish and loose indicating small bowel content.

Colostomies are formed flush to the skin. A single-barrelled colostomy is an end-colostomy, which subsequently forms the end of the alimentary tract. The mobile (transverse and sigmoid) portions of the colon can also be brought out as a loop colostomy. The stoma product is usually firm and brownish suggestive of colonic content.

The site of the stoma does not necessarily dictate whether it's an ileostomy or a colostomy.

CLINICAL

The gentleman in this scenario had Crohn's colitis. How is this differentiated from ulcerative colitis?

Both are forms of inflammatory bowel disease (IBD).

In Crohn's, the inflammation is patchy (skip lesions) and occurs throughout the alimentary tract. The inflammation can involve all layers of the bowel wall and thus deep ulceration is possible, as is fistula formation with adjacent structures. The bowel wall is thickened, and may have a 'cobblestone' appearance endoscopically.

In UC, it is typically only the colon and rectum, which is affected (although the so-called 'backwash' ileitis can occur). As such, panproctocolectomy is usually curative, whereas surgical resection in Crohn's is not. The inflammation is continuous and ulceration confined to the musosa.

Many Crohn's patients undergo serial bowel resections. What is the potential side effect of this and how is the risk managed?

The potential risk is short bowel syndrome. This occurs when sufficient length of (usually small) bowel has been resected so as to result in malabsorption. This can result in deficiencies of a number of vitamins and minerals, with a variety of clinical manifestations. Short bowel syndrome can be temporary, as the remaining short bowel can undergo adaptive changes. To manage the risk of developing a small bowel syndrome, resections in Crohn's are typically avoided and limited wherever possible, and where unavoidable the smallest length possible is resected.

What are the risk factors for anastomotic leaks?

There are a number of risk factors for the formation of anastomotic leaks. These can be considered as 'patient ', "pathology related" and 'technical factors'. Patient factors include smoking, diabetes, PVD, history of corticosteroid use, poor nutritional state and anaemia. Pathology related factors include IBD, collagen disorders and autoimmune disease. Technical factors affect the quality of the anastomosis at surgery and during the postoperative period and include the tension across the anastomosis, local infection, and inadequate blood supply to the cut ends of bowel. The site of anastomosis is also a risk factor, with low rectal> right colonic > small bowel anastomoses.

What are POSSUM and P-POSSUM?

POSSUM and P-POSSUM are widely used and well-validated scoring systems used to inform on the risk of operative intervention by estimating the 30-day morbidity and mortality. It stands for Physiological and Operative Severity Score for the enUmeration of Mortality and morbidity. The additional 'P' of P-Possum refers to the Portsmouth modification to the formula in order to more accurately reflect the risk, but uses the same parameters. These are 12 physiological and 6 operative variables and include: age, cardiac and respiratory history, ECG findings, systolic BP, HR, Hb, WBC, Ur, Na, K, GCS, class of operation, number of procedures performed, operative blood loss, presence of peritoneal contamination, presence +/- spread of malignancy, and CEPOD classification.

SUMMARY

Anastomotic leak can be a serious complication after surgeries involving bowel anastomosis. It can present as an emergency with peritonitis. However, it can also present more indolently with prolonged ileus, vague abdominal pain, low grade pyrexia and tachycardia. Localised leaks can often be managed conservatively after diagnosis with CT and/or water-soluble enema. This often involves bowel rest with an NG tube, antibiotics, and drainage of collections.

TOP TIPS

✚ In very unstable patients, as in this scenario, it is often preferable to proceed with laparotomy immediately without delaying for imaging such as CT.

✚ Young patients, and particularly athletes, may have very robust compensatory mechanisms. Be careful not to be falsely reassured by 'only mildly abnormal' vital signs in these patients.

✚ Although in this scenario the patient had not yet been reviewed by a surgeon, pre-emptively informing the anaesthetists and CEPOD theatre staff can save vital time.

CLINICAL

3.2 Post-Op: Confusion

Scenario

A 67-year-old patient on surgical high care underwent hepatic resection for metastatic colorectal cancer 36 hours ago. The operation was difficult and took longer than expected. Initially, the patient recovered well. However, he is now increasingly confused. His last temperature reading was slightly elevated and his oxygen saturations have dropped despite the nurse administering oxygen through nasal cannulae.

What is your differential diagnosis?

This patient is acutely confused postoperatively. Given the slight pyrexia, development of an oxygen requirement and drop in oxygen saturations basal atelectasis, hospital-acquired pneumonia, or hypoventilation leading to hypoxaemia and hypercarbia are the most likely diagnoses. However, other localised infections or systemic sepsis are possible causes of postoperative confusion, as are poorly controlled pain, overmedication with sedative drugs, drug withdrawal or alcohol withdrawal. More unlikely causes could include intraoperative stroke. Electrolyte imbalances, hepatic/renal failure should be excluded in this case. Moreover, postoperative bile leak or bleeding must be excluded in these patients.

A critical postoperative complication related to liver resections is portal vein thrombosis with increased acidaemia and deteriorating liver function tests. This is an emergency necessitating prompt diagnosis and intervention.

How would you acutely manage this patient?

The patient is acutely unwell and should be approached with an ABCDE algorithm. Airway patency should be confirmed and high-flow oxygen delivered via a non-rebreathe mask delivered in the first instance. Saturations should be continually monitored initially. Vascular access should be secured with two large bore cannulae. Any haemodynamic disturbance should prompt administration of intravenous fluids if appropriate. GCS should be recorded and any lateralising signs noted. The wound should be examined for signs of infection. The patient's medication should be reviewed, paying particular attention to potentially sedating drugs, such as regular or PRN opioids, to ensure adequate (but not over-adequate) administration.

What investigations would aid your diagnosis?

Anaphylaxis is a clinical diagnosis.
Bloods: for U&Es, FBC, LFTs, coag, bone profile.
ABG: for respiratory gases, acid base, glucose and lactate.
CXR (+/- AXR): the signs of which may lag so a negative CXR at this stage does not exclude respiratory pathology.

Consider CTAP and liver doppler to assess collection/portal vein thrombosis.

A CXR reveals some basal atelectasis. How would you manage this?

The patient requires adequate oxygen provision titrated to oxygen saturations. Chest physiotherapy is indicated, and between physiotherapy the patient should be encouraged to cough and take deep breaths. An incentive spirometer can be helpful in this regard. If the patient has signs of chest sepsis antibiotics in line with local protocols should be commenced.

What is the role of antibiotics in basal atelectasis?

There is an increased risk of infection in basal atelectasis, so the patient should regularly be monitored for signs of a developing infection and antibiotics prescribed promptly if any develop. However, atelectasis in and of itself is not an indication for antibiotics.

What factors might have contributed to the development of post-op atelectasis in this patient?

There are a number of factors implicated. A general anaesthetic requires muscular relaxation, intubation and ventilation, which has a number of sequelae which collectively contribute to formation of atelectasis. These include surfactant dysfunction and poor ventilation of basal alveoli. In addition, the relative immobility post-operatively would continue to compromise basal ventilation. Specific to his procedure, the incision used in hepatic resection (though there are several possibilities) is likely a large, painful subcostal incision which will further discourage deep breathing.

The patient's U&Es are show below. What abnormality is demonstrated and what are the potential causes?

Na 125	Ur 7.2
K 4.0	Cr 89
	eGFR 90

The biochemistry result demonstrates a hyponatraemia. Hyponatraemia is commonly seen in the postoperative period and could be responsible for his confusion. One potential cause is that anti-diuretic hormone is secreted as part of the physiological 'stress response' to surgery, creating an SIADH and resulting in hyponatraemia. Another common cause, which may act cumulatively with the stress response, is the inappropriate administration of crystalloid postoperatively with too much volume or too little sodium administered (e.g. use of dextrose). Other causes include drugs, unusual losses of sodium/water (such as in postoperative ileus) amongst others, and are traditionally considered under the headings of hypervolaemic hyponatraemia, euvolaemic hyponatraemia, and hypovolaemic hyponatraemia. Pseudohyponatraemia due to hyperlipidaemia or hyperproteinaemia are also possibilities.

CLINICAL

You notice that the prothrombin time has increased dramatically. What could this represent in this patient?

The most common cause of increased PT time amongst hospital inpatients is vitamin K deficiency. However, PT is a sensitive marker of synthetic hepatic function and this patient is post-hepatic resection. As such the rising PT time could indicate Post-hepatectomy liver failure or small-for-size syndrome, which could also explain his confusion.

SUMMARY

Post-operative confusion is a common complication, particularly in the elderly. It has a myriad of potential causes, from the fairly benign through to life threatening. As such, it should always be investigated. Factors or potential causes can include the patient's pre-existing comorbidities, factors from the procedure itself (such as fat embolus after instrumentation of a long bone), the anaesthetic or other drugs (for example overmedication with opioid analgesics), or factors from the post-operative period (such as nosocomial UTI). There may be multiple factors at play.

The elderly and immunosuppressed represent a particularly challenging population. Advanced age is a risk factor for the development of delirium. Similarly, dementia is a risk factor is its own right and furthermore can mask a developing postoperative confusion. The increased likelihood of complex comorbidity and polypharmacy also complicates the picture in the older age-groups. Postoperative confusion is associated with higher postoperative complication rates, increased mortality, increased length of stay, and the potential for incomplete cognitive recovery.

TOP TIPS

➕ 'Delirium' should not be your diagnosis in and of itself. The aetiology underlying the confusion should be sought and treated.

➕ Beware prematurely attributing post-op confusion to an established diagnosis of dementia.

➕ Hypoactive delirium, which present with a quiet, withdrawn, drowsy confused patient can be more subtle than the agitated patient with hyperactive delirium and should not be missed.

3.3 | Post-Op: Low Blood Pressure

Scenario

A 52-year-old female initially presented with gallstone disease and later undergoes an elective laparoscopic cholecystectomy. You are called to see her post-operatively due to increasing abdominal pain. Her blood pressure is consistent with her baseline at 130/80, but you notice she is slightly tachycardic. Three hours later, you are called again as she has become slightly confused. Her pulse rate has increased to 130 and her blood pressure is now 85/55.

What is your differential diagnosis?

This patient is demonstrating signs of shock. There are a number of potential underlying causes. Bleeding leading to haemorrhagic shock is a high possibility. Considering the preceding operation there could have been injury to the biliary tree or liver, or even bowel or vascular injury. Pulmonary embolus must be considered. Though less likely, myocardial infarction should also be considered. Generalised sepsis due to a wound infection or from other nosocomial infections are unlikely possibilities given the immediate postoperative presentation. Local anaesthetic toxicity should always be thought of as well as anaphylaxis.

How would you acutely manage this patient?

This patient is unstable and should be assessed and treated under the ABCDE protocol. Airway patency should be confirmed and high-flow (15L) oxygen applied through a non-rebreathe mask. The patient will require fluid resuscitation and this should ideally be administered through large-bore peripheral cannulae, preferentially sited in a large vein. The initial resuscitation fluid should ideally be a balanced crystalloid solution such as Hartmanns solution or Plasmalyte. These should be administered as boluses followed by reassessment of the patients vital signs, which then guide further treatment. If only transiently responding to crystalloid, administration of blood should be considered early should the clinical signs suggest postoperative bleeding. The abdomen should be assessed for signs of peritonism. The wound sites should be inspected. A urethral catheter may be introduced to allow for monitoring of urine output. It may be prudent to alert the on-call high-care clinician, and the surgical registrar on call should be notified early.

What investigations would aid your diagnosis?

Urine sample: urine pregnancy test should be tested.
Bloods: including U&E, FBC, LFT, clotting studies, amylase should be sent along with a sample for cross-matching, with 4 units matched urgently.
Arterial (or at least venous) blood gases should be sent, informing on lactate, respiratory function, acid-base status, and glucose.
If resources are available, ultrasonography could be used to assess for intra-abdominal fluid (if the patient is stable).

CLINICAL

Depending on how the patient responds to fluid resuscitation, the options for further investigation include plain abdominal and erect chest radiograph potentially followed by computed tomography if the patient is stabilised, or diagnostic laparoscopy or laparotomy if not.

The patient only transiently responds to crystalloid, but subsequently her parameters worsen further. Her pulse rate is 135, blood pressure 80/50, respiratory rate 34. She has a lactate of 3.2 and a haemoglobin of 82 on her ABG. What is the most likely diagnosis?

She is in hypovolaemic shock secondary to haemorrhage, likely either from an abdominal source or from the abdominal wall at the port sites.

What stage of shock is she in?

She is hypotensive and therefore in stage 3-4 shock. Her heart rate of 135 and respiratory rate of 34 place her in stage 3, which is equivalent with 1.5-2l of blood loss.

	I	II	III	IV
Blood Loss (mL)	<750	750-1500	1500-2000	>2000
Circulating Volume Loss (%)	<15%	15-30%	30-40%	>40%
Heart Rate (Bpm)	Normal	100-120	120-140	>140
Systolic Blood Pressure (mm Hg)	Normal	Normal	Decreased	Decreased
Pulse Pressure	Normal/Increased	Decreased	Decreased	Decreased
Urine Output (mL/Hr)	>30	20-30	5-15	Negligible
Respiratory Rate	14-20	20-30	30-40	>35

What treatment is likely to be indicated, and what would you do?

She is likely to need an urgent laparoscopy/laparotomy. I would ensure that the surgical registrar was updated as to the patients' progress, inform the on-call anaesthetist, and book in to the emergency theatre. I would ensure the haematology lab were processing the G&S urgently and consider utilising O negative blood if there was likely to be any delay.

The patient is taken to theatre by the registrar and consultant. The intraoperative findings were of a large amount of blood in the abdominal cavity, which was suctioned out. The source was a bleeding vessel at the anterior abdominal wall, at a port site. Haemostasis was achieved. The patient received all four units of the cross-matched blood and was stabilised as a result.

SUMMARY

Hypotension due to hypovolaemic/haemorrhagic shock is an emergency. Resuscitation should be via the ABCDE approach and initial fluid resuscitation should be with normal saline or a balanced crystalloid such as Hartmanns'. It should be borne in mind that (approximately) only one-third remains in the vascular space, and therefore larger volumes of fluids are required to replace circulating volume. Dextrose solutions or dextrose saline are inappropriate as they freely distribute across all of the fluid compartments. Prompt identification of an underlying cause is imperative. Fluid resuscitation alone is insufficient management of haemorrhagic ,as in this scenario where the patient was returned to theatre.

TOP TIPS

➕ The percentage of blood loss with respect to the stages of shock can be recalled by considering the scoring in a game of tennis: 0-15,15-30,30-40.

➕ Hypotension is a later sign of haemorrhage than many believe; it does not occur until entering class 3 shock.

➕ Tachycardia and a decrease in pulse pressure precede hypotension as an indicator of hypovolaemic/haemorrhagic shock.

CLINICAL

3.4 Post Op: Low Urine Output

Scenario

The surgical F1 calls you for advice regarding a post-operative patient. The 78-year-old gentleman in question underwent a right hemicolectomy for colorectal cancer the previous day, but has been becoming increasingly confused since then. He has a history of type 2 diabetes mellitus, hypertension and heart failure. He weighs 55 kilograms and has passed 70mls of urine via a urethral catheter over the last 4 hours.

What is your differential diagnosis?

The patient has a urine output of 0.32mls kg-1 hr-1. It is possible that this represents post-operative acute kidney injury, and this must be included. The AKI could in turn be due to many potential aetiologies including hypotension due to haemorrhage/hypovolaemia or 'third-spacing' of fluid due to ileus (NB recent bowel surgery), worsening cardiac failure (NB cardiac history) or others. Other possibilities include blocked urethral catheter, pre-existing renal conditions, but it could also simply be a physiological response resulting from the 'stress response' to surgery.

How would you acutely manage this patient?

The patient is becoming confused and has poor renal output. The cause is unclear and the patient should be comprehensively reviewed with an ABCDE approach with a high index of suspicion. Airway patency should be confirmed and high-flow oxygen applied, initially 15l min-1 via a non-rebreathe mask and subsequently titrated to saturations. Breathing and circulation should be assessed for factors potentially underlying poor urine output but also for alternative explanations of his confusion. Vascular access should be secured with large-bore cannulae and fluid resuscitation may be commenced depending on the clinical findings, cautiously, given history of heart failure. The catheter should be flushed and replaced if either not-flushing, or if the flush cannot subsequently be aspirated.

What investigations would aid your diagnosis?

Bloods including U&Es, FBC, bone profile and LFTs
Bladder scan
Urinalysis plus urgent microscopy
Blood gas analysis for acid-base balance, lactate, and rapid information re: electrolytes.

USS urinary system
CXR if suspicion of pulmonary oedema
ECG +/- troponin if suspected to be cardiogenic
Paired urine and serum osmolalities and biochemistry

Describe the classification of renal failure/kidney injury

Renal failure can be classified as acute or chronic, as well as acute-on-chronic, though acute renal failure is now more frequently known as acute kidney injury and chronic renal failure as chronic kidney disease.

The underlying pathology is classified as pre-renal, renal, or post-renal.

Pre-renal failure results from perturbations to the blood flow to the kidney. These causes can further be categorised into local (e.g. renal artery stenosis or renal vein thrombosis) or systemic (e.g hypovolaemia or hypotension due to another cause).

Renal causes relate to pathology of the kidney itself, such as acute tubular necrosis or one of the numerous nephritides.

Post-renal failure relates to obstruction of the urinary tract. Upper urinary tract obstruction (kindyes and ureter) could be intraluminal (e.g. ureteric stones) or extraluminal (eg. Retroperitoneal fibrosis, malignant ureteric compression). Lower urinary tract obstruction could be due to any pathology causing urethral obstruction (eg. Urethral stricture, prostate disease (malignancy, BPH).

The patient's bloods return demonstrating hyperkalaemia. How would you manage this?

Calcium gluconate 10%; 10mls (cardioprotective)
Insulin + dextrose 10 units insulin in 50mls of 50% dextrose (doses may differ between policies)
Nebulised salbutamol
Cardiac monitoring
Serial serum K+ readings

Involve seniors +/- high care early

What are the indications for dialysis in AKI?

Intractable fluid overload/pulmonary oedema
Intractable hyperkalaemia
Severe metabolic acidosis
Uraemic encephalopathy/pericarditis

How do haemodialysis and haemofiltration differ?

Both methods can be performed in the acute setting (in ITU) through wide-bore double lumen central venous catheters. The blood is anticoagulated (usually heparinised) and pumped through the machine, before being returned to the patient.

In haemofiltration, the blood is pumped at pressure through a semipermeable filter. Hydrostatic pressure drives small molecules and water across the membrane to form an ultrafiltrate, which is discarded and replaced with a replace-

CLINICAL

ment fluid.

In haemodialysis, a dialysate fluid runs countercurrent to the flow of blood, separated by a semi-permeable membrane. The relative concentrations of small molecules equilibriate by diffusion.

Both methods can be employed simultaneously, known as haemodiafiltration.

What scoring systems do you know for acute kidney injury?

The RIFLE and AKIN criteria are the most widely used scoring systems. More recently, the Kidney Disease Improving Global Outcomes (KDIGO) classification has been released.

AKIN Criteria	RIFLE Criteria	Using Creatinine	Using Urine output
Stage 1 AKI	Risk	Cr 1.5x baseline	<0.5mlkg-1hr-1 for over 6 hours
Stage 2 AKI	Injury	Cr 2x baseline	<0.5mlkg-1hr-1 for over 12 hours
Stage 3 AKI (NB this also includes any patient on renal replacement therapy)	Failure	Cr 3x baseline	<0.3mlkg-1hr-1 for over 24 hours or anuria for 12 hours.
	Loss (of function)	Loss of function for over 4 weeks	
	End-stage	End-stage renal disease	

The patient is in pain and agitated. You are unable to pass a 12fr catheter. What would you do and how would you escalate the problem? What if nobody was able to attend to assist you?

Initially it is reasonable to try a different size of catheter. Frequently, a larger catheter is easy to pass, but equally it may be worth attempting with a smaller gauge. There may be other catheters available (eg. Tiemann or Coude catheters). If unable, then it is reasonable to escalate to either the surgical or urology registrar, depending on the hospital. If they too are unable to catheterise, then they may be able to insert a suprapubic catheter. Ultimately, if assistance is not going to be timely enough, it is possible to decompress the bladder percutaneously using a needle.

The patient's potassium normalises over a period of hours with repeated treatment, and with intravenous fluids the renal function improves. The high-care team reviewed the patient but he was successfully managed on the ward.

SUMMARY

Oliguria is a commonly encountered clinical problem, and refers to urine output of less than 0.5 mls kg-1 kg-1. It is frequently seen in the postoperative period. The 'stress response' to surgery includes the release of aldosterone (a mineralocorticoid which acts to increase renal retention of sodium and water and promote potassium excretion) and antidiuretic hormone (which increases the permeability of the collecting ducts as well as altering renal handling of urea and sodium). The result is a physiological reduction in urine output. However, pathological causes of reduced urine output are also common in the postoperative period and thus all cases should be investigated. This patient has a number of risk factors for renal disease including diabetes, hypertension and cardiac failure. As well as being risk factors for AKI these indicates the possibility of pre-existing renal disease in this gentleman.

TOP TIPS

➕ Beware patients with a low BMI. They could have a creatinine within the normal range, but vastly elevated from their baseline and therefore representative of kidney injury.

➕ Hyperkalaemia is a medical emergency which can lead to arrythmogenesis. It is a common derangement in oliguric AKI.

➕ There are numerous causes of pseudohyperkalaemia- for example prolonged tourniquet time or use of a small-bore needle at phlebotomy.

CLINICAL

3.5 | Post-Op: Leg Swelling

Scenario

As the on-call orthopaedic core surgical trainee, you have been called to review a 67-year-old gentleman with right sided leg and calf swelling, seven days following a right sided total knee replacement for osteoarthritis.

What is your differential diagnosis?

- DVT
- Post-Op haemarthrosis and oedema
- Infection
- Lymphoedema
- Fracture

All surgical patients are at risk of developing deep vein thrombosis (DVT). Those who have assisted in total knee arthroplasty surgery will note that most surgeons deflate the tourniquet once the wound has been closed and the dressings have been applied. It is not uncommon for the knee to be 'oozy' from the bony cuts and soft tissue dissection and so once the tourniquet has been deflated, the joint can fill up with haemarthrosis. It is expected that these patients will have some elements of knee swelling post operation around the joint and operative site and this can be addressed by simple maneuvers such as elevating the limb as well as applying cryotherapy (ice). The latter also aids in addressing postoperative pain.

Another differential diagnosis is a postoperative infection, but given the relative short time from surgery, this diagnosis is unlikely. Routine bloods would reveal increased inflammatory markers and so you cannot rely on the inflammatory markers for the diagnosis. This diagnosis must be based on the clinical presentation.

How would you acutely manage this patient?

All surgically unwell patients must be assessed and managed according to the ABCDE approach, as taught on the CCrISP and ATLS courses. Immediate symptomatic management such as pain relief would allow for an accurate assessment, allowing you to implement interventions tailored to your examination findings.

Once you have administered analgesia, assessed the patient through the ABCDE approach, you must focus your examination on the knee. All joint examinations follow the Look, Feel and Move approach. Therefore, you must assess the amount of swelling, its location, condition of the surrounding skin and state of the wound. Ensure that the dressings are taken down and be sure to wear gloves. You may also ask the nursing staff as to whether they have changed the dressings already, and if they have, how soaked they were with blood?

You should palpate the knee joint for warmth (which it would be post-operation), and any tenderness (which again may be the case post-operation). Then you ask the patient to move the limb to full extension and then full flexion. Most patients at this stage would only bear 0 degrees extension to 90 degrees of flexion. However, if there is significant swelling, the patient may not have an impressive range of motion due to a tense haemarthrosis. Complete your examination by assessing the limbs neurovascular status.

Finally, enquire as to whether the patient had DVT prophylaxis such as LMWH and TED Stockings and review the notes (surgical operation note, in patient notes and the drug charts).

What investigations would aid your diagnosis?

Bloods: FBC and CRP may be raised post operation so this should be interpreted cautiously. Moreover, a D-Dimer will also be raised. The biochemical profile should be completed by obtaining U&Es as well as obtaining the coagulation profile of the patient.

Blood Cultures: If the temperature is raised or you suspect an infected joint, take blood cultures and speak to the operating surgeon prior to commencing antibiotics.

Radiograph: A post-operation, check radiograph should already have been performed so review that. If the clinical presentation warrants, you can repeat the AP and lateral radiograph of the post-operative knee which may reveal a fracture, which is another cause for swelling in the knee.

Duplex USS: Finally, if you are suspicious of a DVT, then start therapeutic LMWH and obtain a duplex ultra sound scan.

Do you know any scoring system for DVT? What is its purpose?

The Wells' score is used to assess the clinical probability of a DVT.

What are the clinical features of deep vein thrombosis?

This is encompassed in the Wells' score, shown below. This can help you predict clinically the likelihood of a DVT.

Clinical Feature	Points
Active Cancer (treatment ongoing, within 6 months, or palliative	1
Paralysis, paresis or recent plaster immobilization of the lower extremities	1
Recently bedridden for 3 days or more or major surgery within 12 weeks requiring general or regional anaesthesia	1
Localised tenderness along the distribution of the deep venous system	1
Entire leg swollen	1
Calf swelling at least 3 cm larger than asymptomatic side	1

Pitting oedema confined to the symptomatic leg	1
Collateral superficial veins (non-varicose)	1
Previously documented DVT	1
An alternative diagnosis is at least as likely as DVT	-2

If DVT is considered 'likely':

- Patient should have d-dimer, and
- Duplex leg veins within 4 hours.
- *(If unable to perform within 4 hours, to have scan in 24 hours with interim dose of parenteral anticoagulant).*
- If d-dimer is positive and the duplex is negative, a repeat duplex is recommended in one week.

If DVT is considered 'unlikely':

- Patient should have d-dimer.
- If positive – for duplex leg veins within 4 hours.
- If unable to perform within 4 hours, to have scan in 24 hours with interim dose of parenteral anticoagulant.

It should be noted that Well's score is ultimately an aid to diagnosis, and should be balanced with the level of clinical suspicion for the specific patient. Imaging should be considered for cases with high suspicion of DVT regardless of score.

This gentleman is deemed to have high risk for DVT and you therefore arranged duplex for his deep venous system, which has returned confirming a proximal DVT. How would you manage this?

For a confirmed DVT, patients should be anticoagulated with low molecular weight heparin (LMWH) provided that there are no contraindications. Oral anticoagulants, such as warfarin or novel oral anticoagulants (NOACs) should be started at the same time after consulting your local hospital departmental guide. Upon satisfactory loading of oral anticoagulants, the LMWH can be stopped. This is usually determined by the anticoagulation team, so ensure that you have consulted them also.

The duration of treatment for unprovoked DVT would be at least 3 months; further discussion should take place with the patient with regards to extending anticoagulation for a further 3 months.

Iliofemoral DVT may require a referral to the vascular surgeons for consideration of catheter-directed thrombolytic therapy or mechanical thrombectomy. If the patient is unable to receive anticoagulation medical, a temporary inferior vena caval filter could be offered to prevent secondary pulmonary embolism from a dislodged clot from the leg.

Further investigation for the cause of DVT/PE should be considered if no obvious cause is found. In this case the patient has surgery as the reasonable

CLINICAL

cause of his DVT. However, if he develops another DVT, then it may be necessary to investigate him further for a cause i.e. thrombophiliac screen +/- referral
to haematologist.

What complications would this gentleman be at risk of as a consequence of his DVT?

This gentleman would be at risk of pulmonary embolism. Further complications
such as post-thrombotic syndrome can occur with symptoms including pain,
swelling, haemosiderin deposition and varicose veins. In severe cases this can
lead to venous ulceration. Prevention and treatment strategies include eleva-
tion, compression stockings and early mobilisation.

SUMMARY

Deep vein thrombosis is a relatively common complication of total knee replacement. Common presenting features include unilateral leg swelling with pitting
oedema. There may be tenderness along the distribution of the deep venous
system. Due to the blockage of the deep system, collateral superficial varicosi-
ties may be seen on examination. Investigation should be directed according
to Wells score with d-dimer and duplex of the deep venous system. Treatment
involves anticoagulation for 3-6 months. Post-thrombotic syndrome is a long
term and serious complication of deep vein thrombosis.

TOP TIPS

CLINICAL

➕ DVT post total knee replacement can be a consequence and a
cause of a downward spiral of immobility and stiffness. Prompt
intervention is key.

➕ Perioperative VTE prophylaxis *(pneumatic pump, perioperative
hydration)* is a commonly forgotten aspect of the overall VTE
prevention strategy.

➕ Vascular opinion should be sought for iliofemoral DVT as there
may be a need for catheter-directed thrombolytic therapy or mechanical thrombectomy. SVC filter can be considered if anticoagulation is contraindicated.

3.6 Post-Op: Tonsillar Bleed

Scenario

A 22-year-old patient presents to A&E 24 hours after having had a bilateral tonsillectomy with worsening pain, bleeding from the mouth, tachycardia, pyrexia and has not eaten or drank anything since discharge yesterday.

What is your differential diagnosis?

Post-tonsillectomy bleed, caused by lack of haemostasis in theatre.
Not eating and drinking post operation.
Infection (less likely to be the cause within 48 hours of the operation).
Other differentials could include haemoptysis or upper GI bleed.

How would you acutely manage this patient?

I would stabilise the patient using an ABCDE approach and immediately put oxygen on the patient (15L non rebreathe mask) and assess his airway. He most likely will need suction to help clear his airway. I would place a saturation monitor on him, listen to his chest, and check for equal air expansion to assess his breathing. If A and B were stable, I would move on to C where I would ensure adequate IV access by inserting two large bore cannulae. At the same time I would send bloods for FBC, U&Es, clotting screen and a group and save or cross match depending on how much he was bleeding. I would assess his blood pressure, heart rate and capillary refill and give Hartmann's IV if this was low via fluid boluses. I would ensure my seniors are informed early as this patient may need to go back to theatre for surgical management. I would insert a catheter if it was a large bleed to monitor fluid balance, administer IV antibiotics according to trust policy (usually benzylpenicillin and metronidazole) and give adequate analgesia. I would then reassess.

What investigations would aid your diagnosis?

Bloods: FBC, U&Es, clotting and G&S
You may need to use a fine nasoendoscope if concerned about other causes of bleeding in the throat.

You call the on call ENT registrar but he is 30 minutes away from the hospital, your patient is still bleeding from the mouth, how would you stop this bleeding?

First I would examine the tonsillar fossa to look for any bleeding points. I would use a local anaesthetic spray with adrenaline in and also try to cauterise any bleeding vessels using a silver nitrate stick. If there were

CLINICAL

no obvious bleeding points I would ask the patient to gargle hydrogen peroxide 3% diluted 1:4.

You have halted the bleeding slightly but the bleeding may start again, what else could you do before the registrar arrives?

 Keeping the patient nil by mouth, I would optimise the patient for theatre. I would inform the anaesthetists and theatre staff that there may be a patient for theatre who is bleeding. I would ensure all correct documentation was in place and I would consent the patient if I felt competent to do this.

If this patient had only had a small bleed, spitting out less than a teaspoon of blood which had stopped and on examination you can see a small clot in the tonsillar fossa, how would your management differ?

 I would still use an ABCDE approach, bloods, cannula and IV antibiotics and fluids. I would still admit them for observations as a small bleed can precede a large haemorrhage (a heralding bleed). At this time the patient would most likely not require full fluid resuscitation and catheterisation.

If this patient was day 5 post-operation what is the most likely cause?

This would be a secondary bleed and the most likely cause would be an infection and the patient not eating and drinking well post-op.

SUMMARY

The risk of a post tonsillectomy bleed within the first 24 hours is about 1-2%. A secondary tonsillar bleed occurs around 5-9 days post-op and is most likely due to infection in the slough on the tonsils that hasn't been removed if the patient isn't eating and drinking. The patient could also present like an epistaxis if they have had an adenoidectomy – management principles are the same.

TOP TIPS

 Know how to initially manage any bleeding patient using the ABCDE approach.

 Understand that any post-tonsillectomy bleed is significant.

CLINICAL

3.7 | Post-Op: Paraphimosis

Scenario

You are called to see a 72-year-old gentleman on one of the orthopaedic wards who is becoming increasingly agitated. He underwent a cemented hemiarthroplasy under spinal anaesthesia on the trauma list earlier in the day. He is complaining of pain and keeps pulling at the urinary catheter, which was inserted immediately prior to his operation.

What is your differential diagnosis?

UTI
Post-op agitation
Paraphimosis
Urinary retention/injury

It is possible that in the immediate post-op period the patient is confused/re-covering and is alarmed at having a catheter in situ, however, this should be a diagnosis of exclusion. Paraphimosis is a likely cause of penile/suprapubic pain after a recent catheterisation in a male. He could be experiencing suprapubic pain in response to a urinary tract infection introduced by catheterisation, or another genital infection such as epididymitis- although the time period is too brief for this. He could be agitated and in pain from urinary retention caused by a blockage in the catheter. There may have been complication with catheter insertion, including urethral injury from traumatic passage or premature inflation of the balloon, creation of a false passage, or sensitivity/allergy to the substance of the catheter itself.

How would you acutely manage a patient with a paraphimosis?

Although this is likely the source of the patients agitation, he is nonetheless agitated post-operatively therefore the patient should receive an ABCDE assessment to ensure there was no other pathology and that the patient is stable.

Presuming that he is, it should be ensured that the patient is prescribed appropriate analgesia and that this is appropriately administered. The catheter and bag should be quickly checked to ensure it has been draining adequate amounts of urine. However, paraphimosis is a urological emergency and therefore the main priority would be to attempt manual reduction. If unable to reduce the paraphimosis, urgent urological opinion should be sought. It is also important to assess the skin for necrosis or cellulitis which can complicate a long-standing paraphimosis.

Describe the technique for simple manual reduction of a paraphimosis

The area should be cleaned and draped, and appropriate protective wear donned. The glans and oedematous foreskin are initially compressed for a number of minutes in a bid to manually alleviate some of the swelling. After this, the thumbs are placed side-by-side on the glans, and the index fingers placed behind the incarcerated prepuce. The reduction is a gradual process of pressure from the thumbs, to further reduce the swelling, and gentle traction with the fingers upon the foreskin. The trick is to ensure that the phimotic band is pulled back over the glans as it is this, which causes the preputial oedema. Simply pulling the swollen foreskin back over the glans will not resolve the condition.

What are the pathophysiological sequence of events which lead to the formation of a paraphimosis?

In paraphimosis, the prepuce remains retracted proximal to the corona of the glans penis and forms a constricting ring at this point. This initially impedes lymphatic and venous return, causing engorgement of the vessels distal to the paraphimosis and oedema of the glans and of the retracted prepuce itself. The swelling then leads to a worsening of the obstruction to lymphatic and venous return, further worsening venocongestion and oedema.

What are the potential sequelae if left untreated?

If left untreated, the paraphimosis eventually leads to ischaemia of the affected tissues by affecting the arterial supply. Like a compartment syndrome, the interstitial pressure distal to the tourniquet effect of the paraphimosis increases and reduces the perfusion pressure of the affected parts of the penis. The clinical result is necrosis, and eventually autoamputation, of the penis.

You are unable to reduce the paraphimosis. The on-call urologist attends but prior to attempting further reduction wishes for greater analgesia. He opts for regional local anaesthesia. What regional block will he perform and how is it performed?

If the patient has not received sufficient analgesia from parenteral analgesia, then a penile block under local anaesthesia can be beneficial. It involves anaesthetising the two dorsal penile nerves (right and left). These are located at the ten and two o'clock positions (assuming 12 o'clock is caudad). This should be performed as proximally as possible. Alternatively, a circumferential approach, injecting small amounts of anaesthetic circumferentially about the base of the penis can be used.

What common addition to local anaesthetic must you ensure is absent and why?

The local anaesthetic must not contain adrenaline. Adrenaline is commonly added as a vasoconstrictor to potentiate the anaesthetic effects. However, it is absolutely contraindicated in areas with end-arterial supply such as digits or the penis. In paraphimosis, the distal perfusion is already compromised, making this even more vital than it would be otherwise.

CLINICAL

What other non-operative techniques could be used to reduce this paraphimosis?

The osmotic method involves bathing the penis in a concentrated solution (or wrapping it in swabs bathed in the solution) for example 50% dextrose. The concept is that this draws the fluid from the oedema by osmosis, facilitating reduction.

Another method, known as the Dundee technique, can also be used. This involves making a number of punctures with a needle into the oedematous prepuce which allows the escape of the oedema fluid in response to pressure. Manual traction can then be reattempted.

How is the condition managed in children?

Paraphimosis can occur in children. The main difficulty is managing an often worried child and parents. Analgesic options may also be limited. If a manual reduction is not successful or tolerated then have a low threshold for performing reduction under a brief general anaesthetic in theatre.

SUMMARY

Paraphimosis is a urological emergency, and occurs when the retracted prepuce progressively obstructs vascular return from the distal penis resulting in pain and swelling. Prompt resolution is required as untreated, it can go on to obstruct the arterial supply. This is in contrast to a phimosis, which is an inability to retract the foreskin and is often physiological, particularly in children. Paraphimosis is most commonly iatrogenic, but can also occur in the context of trauma, vigorous sexual activity, infection, or forceful retraction of a phimosis.

CLINICAL

TOP TIPS

➕ Paraphimosis is usually painful and this may be the presenting feature. However, beware instances when this is not the case. For example, the patient in this scenario had recent spinal anaesthesia, which could have masked this paraphimosis developing.

➕ It is crucial to replace the prepuce after urethral catheterisation and to document this in the medical notes,

➕ If concerned or unable to reduce the paraphimosis, early urological consultation is vital due to the sequelae if left untreated.

3.8 | Post-Op: Temperature

Scenario

You are the general surgical CT1 on call and have been asked to review a 65-year-old gentleman who has spiked a temperature of 38.3 8-days post-op, following an elective open anterior resection for bowel cancer. He is tachypnoeic (RR 24) and tachycardic (116 bpm).

What is your differential diagnosis?

Infectious causes with SIRS response
- Wound infection *(superficial or deep)*
- Intra-abdominal collection
- Anastomotic leak
- Nosocomial infection - hospital acquired pneumonia, ventilator associated pneumonia, urinary tract infection, MRSA, Clostridium Difficile
- Aspiration pneumonia *(Mendelson's syndrome)*
- Device related infection – peripheral or central line infection, urinary catheter

Non-infectious causes
- Drug induced fever
- Venous thromboembolism
- Physiological response to surgical trauma
- Atelectasis
- Pain
- Occult Haemorrhage
- Non-haemolytic febrile related transfusion reaction *(if transfused)*

How would you manage the patient?

The patient should be stabilised following an ABCDE approach and because this gentleman is septic you should treat as per the sepsis six guidelines:

Airway: Check airway is patent
Breathing: Note oxygen saturations and RR (check the trend). Apply 15L/minute oxygen via a non-rebreathe mask and adequately expose and examine the chest: any use of the accessory muscles? Any evidence of respiratory distress? Symmetrical breathing? Equal chest expansion? Trachea central? Percuss the chest and auscultate (anterior and posterior)
Circulation: Get IV access with two large-bore cannulas and take bloods at this time (FBC, U/Es, CRP, LFTs, Clotting, Amylase, Blood Cultures, Group and Save), check HR and BP and note the trend. Check capillary refill time, listen to heart sounds, check JVP and ask for a 12-lead ECG and asses for any evidence of peripheral oedema

CLINICAL

Fluid resuscitation

 I would like to review notes/ask the patient if he has any known cardiac history. If no cardiac history and not clinically overloaded I would trial with a 500ml bolus of Hartmann's initially and reassess; if known cardiac history I would resuscitate more cautiously and give a 250ml bolus of Hartmann's. I would titrate fluids to patient response and correction of haemodynamic parameters.

Disability: GCS/AVPU, check blood glucose and pupils (size/equal?)

Exposure: Expose the patient appropriately and examine as required Review the drug chart. Review analgesia requirements and administer analgesia if the patient is in pain. Has all medication prescribed been administered (e.g. antibiotics, anticoagulants).

Review the operation note: Is there an anastomosis? Any complications in surgery?

Review the patient's notes: Is this an acute deterioration? How has the patient been post-op? Other comorbidities?

Sepsis Six: The gentleman will also need urinary catheterisation as per Sepsis Six Pathway and monitor response to fluids. Check urine analysis when catheterised. Antibiotics should be given as per Trust Protocol and Sepsis Six Pathway within 1 hour of diagnosis.

If at any stage you have any concerns make sure you seek senior help.

What investigations would you order?

12-Lead ECG: to assess tachycardia and exclude any acute ischaemic events

Bloods: baseline, CRP, blood cultures and ABG

Cultures: of any peripheral/central lines

Urine dipstick: to assess for urinary tract infection. Send for MC&S if positive.

CXR: to assess if are any areas of opacification suggestive of infection or fluid overload

USS abdomen: any free fluid or collections?

CT Abdomen Pelvis: (with contrast if renal function within acceptable range) to assess for free peritoneal fluid, presence, site and size of abscess. This will be used to direct operative management.

A CT scan was performed which shows evidence of an intra-abdominal abscess. What is the diagnosis and would your long-term management be?

The combination of clinical signs and investigations are indicative of an anastomotic leak resulting in peritonitis with intra-abdominal abscess formation. Initial management should be as per the sepsis six pathway, ensuring close monitoring and titrating to patient response and observations.

Depending on the clinical state of the patient they may need to go to theatre urgently, or a trial of IV broad spectrum antibiotics and resuscitation may be appropriate and if no improvement the patient will then need emergency surgery to manage infection.

What is the definite management of an intra-abdominal abscess?

Following the surgical dictum "Ubi pus, ibi evacua" (where there is pus, evacuate it) the treatment of an abscess requires drainage. The ideal management should follow a multi-disciplinary approach involving members such as a surgeon, radiologist, specialist colorectal nurse and specialist stoma care nurse to plan the appropriate option for each individual case. Options may include image-guided percutaneous drainage (ultrasound or CT-guided), or surgical drainage through single or multi-staged approaches.

Are you aware of any scoring systems to predict risk of surgery?

The Physiological and Operative Severity Score for the enumeration of Mortality and Morbidity (POSSUM) score was developed in 1991 by Copeland et al and revised in 1998 as the Portsmouth POSSUM (P-POSSUM) score. It is commonly used by surgeons in the UK to estimate risk of mortality for patients undergoing surgery and has been adapted for different specialities: P-POSSUM for general surgery, CR-POSSUM for colorectal surgery, Vascular-POSSUM for vascular surgery, O-POSSUM for oesophagogastric. The possum score takes into consideration both physiological and operative factors

The patient has an INR of 2.5 as he has had his warfarin re-started post-op. He takes warfarin for a metallic heart valve. What would you give him to acutely reduce his INR?

Given that his warfarin is for a metallic heart valve you should speak with the cardiologists and follow local trust guidelines to safely reduce his risk of intraoperative bleeding. Typically this involves slowly reversing his warfarin with oral vitamin K while covering his metallic valve risk with heparin. In any patient with a high bleeding risk fresh frozen plasma (FFP) can be given pre or intra-op to reverse clotting abnormalities. Trusts have varying protocols for reversal of clopidogrel and novel oral anticoagulants (NOACs) such as dabigatran.

What are the differences between SIRS, sepsis and septic shock?

SIRS is the symptoms and signs of infection.
The patient needs to have two of the following: temperature >38 degrees or < 36 degrees, tachycardia > 90bpm, tachypnoea >20, WCC >12 or <4, altered mental state and a BM >6.6.
Sepsis is SIRS with a confirmed infection and severe sepsis is sepsis with altered organ perfusion or dysfunction.
Septic shock is refractory hypotension is addition to severe sepsis.

What is sepsis six?

Sepsis six is from the 'surviving sepsis campaign'.
It is the evidence behind improving survival rates with sepsis by optimising the treatment given within the first 6 hours of symptoms.
It includes giving high flow oxygen, taking blood cultures, giving antibiotics, IV fluids, checking Hb and lactate levels, and measuring hourly urine outputs.

CLINICAL

SUMMARY

This scenario involved a post-operative anastomotic leak following colorectal surgery, presenting with signs of sepsis through a positive systemic inflammatory response. This can lead to intra-abdominal abscesses which are typically polymicrobial, containing both gram negative and anaerobic organisms. The definitive treatment is drainage of the abscess and repair of the anastomotic leak which may require a multi-stage approach.

TOP TIPS

✚ Have a high index of suspicion of anastomic leak in patients post-colorectal surgery who develop SIRS response.

✚ It is important to manage the patient using an ABCDE approach and consider the multiple causes of the SIRS response.

✚ POSSUM scores are useful to calculate the risk of mortality for patients who require surgery.

CLINICAL

3.9 | Upper GI Bleed

Scenario

A dishevelled 63-year-old male presents acutely with a four-hour history of abdominal pain and 'coffee ground' vomit. This has coincided with a one-week history of loose stool that is black and foul smelling. Examination reveals significant epigastic rebound and percussion tenderness with no evidence of peritonism. His bowel sounds are audible. Digital rectal exam reveals black loose stool on the tip of the glove. He is tacchycardic (110bpm) and hypotensive (90/60) on presentation.

What is your differential diagnosis?

Oesophageal varices: the patient's 'dishevelled' appearance may point towards chronic alcohol abuse.
Common causes: Mallory-Weiss tear (often associated with repeated bouts of vomiting), peptic ulceration, oesophagitis, gastritis, duodenitis, drugs (e.g. NSAIDs, aspirin), idiopathic.
Rare causes: bleeding disorders, angiodysplasia, portal hypertensive gastropathy, aorto-enteric fistula, Peutz-Jeghers' syndrome.

How would you acutely manage this patient?

Adopting an ABCDE approach is vital with protection of the airway and high flow oxygen given if required. Patients with fluctuating conscious levels are at risk of aspiration. IV access gained via two large-bore cannulae within the ante-cubital fossae. Fluid resuscitation should be titrated to patient response if there is any suspicion of heamodynamic compromise. Crystalloid should be used in the early stages before cross-matched blood becomes available however if the patient continues to bleed, O Rh-ve blood should be considered.

A catheter should also be inserted as an hourly urine output provides a useful measure of hydrational status. Analgesia should be administered to ensure the patient is comfortable. A CVP line may be used to monitor and give fluid replacement. IV PPI (e.g. IV omeprazole 40mg) may be considered AFTER endoscopy (reduces the risk of rebleeding and need for surgery, but not mortality, in peptic ulcer bleeding).
Once the patient is stabilised a comprehensive history and examination should be conducted to identify the underlying cause. Inform your senior early including making ITU/HDU aware of the patient.

What investigations would aid your diagnosis?

Bloods: FBC (Hb may be normal in acute blood loss), U&Es (a raised urea:creatinine ration points to a large blood meal), LFTs, clotting, CRP, ESR, group and save, X-matching, ABG.
Radiographs: If perforation is suspected an erect CXR and AXR may be useful to identify free-air.

CLINICAL

Endoscopy: should be arranged within four hours. This can be used to diagnose and treat (including banding/sclerotherapy) as well as identify risk of further bleeding.

CT angiography: provides a non-invasive means to identify source of bleeding however this is not often requested in the acute phase.

What clinical signs on examination might indicate a provisional diagnosis of variceal bleeding?

Look for evidence of chronic liver disease, these include: splenomegaly, encephalopathy, coagulopathy, thrombocytopenia, ascites and hyponaetremia. You could also screen for signs of alcohol abuse including hair loss and peripheral neuropathy.

What risk-scoring system do you know for upper GI bleeds?

The Rockall scoring. The scoring system is used to predict rebleeding risk and mortality following an upper GI bleed. A score of greater than 6 often warrants urgent surgical intervention however decisions for surgery are rarely taken on the basis of the score alone.

	0	1	2	3
PRE-ENDOSCOPY				
Age (yrs)	<60	60-79	>80	
BP (sys)	No shock	BP>100	BP<100	
HR (bpm)		HR>100		
Co-morbidity	Nil major	Cardiac failure, ischaemic heart disease	Renal/liver failure	Metastases
POST-ENDOSCOPY				
Diagnosis		Mallory-Weiss tear, no lesion.	Other diagnosis	Upper GI malignancy
Signs of recent haemorrhage on endoscopy		None		Blood in upper GI tract

What are the indications for surgery in upper GI bleeds?

Severe bleeding or bleeding despite transfusing > 6 units if over 60 years and >8 units of blood if under 60 years.

Other indications include uncontrollable bleeding at endoscopy, rebleeding, or a Rockhall score ≥3 initially or final >6.

What are the common sites for variceal formation?

Varices most commonly occur in the lower oesophagus, but are also found in the greater curvature of the stomach, rectum as well as around the umbilicus (caput medusae).

What are the commonly used treatment modalities for bleeding varices in an acute setting?

Starting IV Terlipressin early with a 2mg bolus helps to reduce the risk of death. Endoscopy provides an opportunity to use banding or sclerotherapy however in cases of uncontrolled bleeding a Sengstaken-Blakemore tube may be inflated to tamponade the site of bleeding.

What treatment methods are used to limit the risk of variceal re-bleeding?

The risk of further variceal bleeding after the initial bleed can be as high as 80% within the first two years. Non-selective beta-blockade (e.g.propanolol 40-80mg) can be used with repeat endoscopic band ligation another option. In patients who are resistant to band therapy, transjugular intrahepatic portosystemic shunting (TIPPS) can be used to redirect blood away from the liver by connecting the portal and hepatic veins in the liver.

SUMMARY

Melaena (black, tar coloured stool) as well as coffee ground vomit are symptoms of partially digested blood, both indicative of upper GI bleeding. Your initial examination provides vital clues to the initial aetiology. For example hepatic decompensation as a result of chronic alcohol abuse can manifest with distinctive signs and symptoms. Initial treatment is aimed at attempting to restore heamodynamic status, with endoscopy used to identify and treat the likely source of bleeding.

Variceal bleeding has a high risk of reoccurrence and mortality can be predicted by using the Rockhall score. Banding and sclerotherapy form the main means of intervention however a Sengstaken-Blakemore tube can also be used in treatment resistant cases.

CLINICAL

TOP TIPS

✚ Early fluid resuscitation and escalation to your senior is vitally important in patients who demonstrate hypovolaemic compromise.

✚ In suspected variceal bleeding sclerotherapy and endoscopic band ligation form the main means of surgical intervention.

✚ Risk of rebleeding is extremely high and therefore prophylactic measures with active surveillance must be adopted.

3.10 Abdominal Distension

Scenario

A 72-year-old morbidly obese male presents acutely with a six-day history of progressive abdominal distension and absolute constipation. He now complains of generalised abdominal discomfort and nausea. His past medical history includes type II diabetes mellitus controlled with insulin, angina and a previous left inguinal hernia repair. Examination reveals a non-tender abdomen, which is grossly distended. There is no guarding or rebound tenderness. He is afebrile and normotensive, with a heart rate of 102 bpm.

What is your differential diagnosis?

Large bowel obstruction: this is most likely as symptoms of constipation and progressive abdominal distension precede nausea. An absence of early vomiting also points away from a small bowel obstruction. Although hernias and adhesions secondary to intrabdominal surgery are common causes of small bowel obstruction – the site of hernia repair in this case makes large bowel obstruction more likely.
Small bowel obstruction, pseudo-obstruction (Ogilvie's syndrome), ileus.

How would you acutely manage this patient?

A conventional ABCDE approach should be used to stabilise the patient in an acute setting. A 'drip and suck' method is usually adopted where intravenous crystalloids are given and any electrolyte abnormalities corrected. An NGT should be inserted to allow the stomach to decompress.

A catheter should also be inserted as urine output provides an early measure of hydrational status. The patient should be kept nil by mouth, with maintenance fluids prescribed. Ideally your senior colleagues should be informed early as the patient may require surgical intervention.

Once the patient is stabilised a comprehensive history and examination should be conducted to identify the underlying cause.

What investigations would aid your diagnosis?

Bloods: FBC, U&Es, LFTs, clotting, CRP, ESR, group and save, cross-matching, VBG (to assess lactate)
AXR: site, diameter as well as presence of haustra help to distinguish between large and small bowel. Dilated bowel loops often conform to the rule of three (>3cm = small bowel, >6cm = large bowel, >9cm = caecum). The presence of air within the abdomen (e.g. Rigler's sign) is indicative of perforation.
Erect CXR: screen for air under the diaphragm (sign of bowel perforation).
Colonoscopy: may be warranted in cases of mechanical intraluminal obstruction however there is a risk of perforation.

Water soluble contrast (e.g. Gastrografin study): helpful in determining the level of obstruction with mild therapeutic benefit.

CT abdomen: demonstrates the transition point of obstruction clearly as well as the likely cause.

What abnormal gas patterns are indicative of bowel perforation in an erect CXR and AXR?

An erect CXR helps delineate any free air within the abdomen which rises and can be seen underneath the diaphragm. An AXR may demonstrate free air outside of the bowel wall. Rigler's sign may be present where both sides of the bowel wall are seen with distinct triangular shaped segments. A sharp liver edge may also be present.

How would you further investigate and manage the patient in an acute setting?

Contacting the senior registrar early in this case is essential. A comprehensive history and examination should be conducted to identify a root cause for the obstruction. Constipation is more likely to be absolute if the obstruction is distal. Tinkling bowel sounds may be ascultated. Fermentation of the intestinal contents may produce faecal vomiting and often occurs where there is a colonic fistula in the proximal gut.

The majority of patients with a sigmoid volvulus can be managed by passing a rigid sigmoidoscope with the patient in a lateral position. This allows for bowel decompression, with the patient monitored in the following days for bowel ischaemia or necrosis.

What group of patients are susceptible to a sigmoid volvulus?

The condition tends to occur in elderly patients who suffer from chronic constipation with numerous comordities and poor mobility. It is responsible for 8% of bowel obstructions.

What are the other common causes of large bowel obstruction?

Common causes include constipation, hernias, adhesions secondary to intrabdominal surgery, and tumours. Less common causes include intussusception (paediatric cases), gallstone ileus, Crohn's disease, diverticular strictures, and a foreign body.

How would you proceed if your initial conservative management strategy fails?

With raised inflammatory markers and high lactate the patient may be developing critical bowel ischaemia secondary to sigmoid torsion. This has a high risk of progressing to necrosis without surgical intervention. Informing your senior early as well as optimising the patient preoperatively including cross-matching 4 units of blood is required. A rectal tube is inserted to evacuate the sigmoid contents, and a lower midline incision performed with the redundant sigmoid loop resected and immediate anatomises or colostomy carried out.

CLINICAL

SUMMARY

Sigmoid volvulus occurs when the bowel twists on its mesentery, which can rapidly progress to strangulation. There are numerous predisposing factors however the condition can often arise with no underlying cause. Insertion of a NGT to aid decompression is vital as simply placing the patient nil by mouth does nothing to rest the bowel, which produces over 9 litres of fluid per day. Acute strangulation or closed loop obstruction are indicators for immediate surgery and hence should be escalated early. Conservative measures including passing a rigid sigmoidoscope should be trialled first as the majority of cases resolve following this intervention.

TOP TIPS

➕ Strangulated bowel can manifest rapidly once a sigmoid volvulus has occurred resulting in tissue necrosis. This is therefore a surgical emergency.

➕ A characteristic 'U' or 'coffee-bean' shape is seen on the AXR.

➕ It tends to occur in elderly patients with multiple-comorbidites and is often managed with a rigid sigmoidoscope and insertion of a flatus tube.

CLINICAL

3.11 | Erythema

Scenario

A 35-year-old intravenous drug user presented a few days after injecting heroin into his right groin with severe pain around the injection site. The patient is unwell with a low urine output. Clinically, erythema extends to the right flank and medial thigh. There is oedema extending beyond the site of erythema with associated blisters and crepitus noted on palpation.

What is your differential diagnosis?

Necrotising fasciitis
Cellulitis and abscess
Infected arterio-venous fistula
Strangulated femoral hernia

How would you acutely manage this patient?

Primary survey
Airway assessment and oxygenation
Breathing and ventilation
Circulation: fluid resuscitation, catheterise and monitor fluid output. Send off blood tests including cross match.
Disability: GCS assessment and check blood glucose
Exposure: examine with preservation of dignity and prevention of hypothermia.

Secondary survey
AMPLE history
Full examination

Commence sepsis bundle
Start intravenous antibiotics after discussion with the microbiologists
Recognise the need for emergency surgical intervention:

- Inform the senior surgical team
- Inform the ITU for admission
- Inform the on call anaesthetist and emergency theatre coordinator
- Prepare the patient for theatres for emergency debridement

What investigations would aid your diagnosis?

Bloods: elevated WBC, CRP and creatine kinase, arterial blood gases and blood cultures
Imaging: Xray, USS, CT or MRI will show air in subcutaneous tissue and exclude other differential diagnoses.

CLINICAL

What are the types of necrotising fasciitis?

Type I: Polymicrobial infection (aerobic and anaerobic bacteria) or atypical bacterium.

Type II: Secondary to haemolytic Group A Streptococcus (e.g. Strep Pyogenes) +/ coexisting staphylococcal infection.

Type III: Gas gangrene, caused by Clostridium Perfringens or less commonly Clostridia Septicum.

Name any special tests in aiding your diagnosis of necrotising fasciitis

The 'finger sweep test': when necrotising fasciitis is suspected, an incision can be made over the suspected area. Presence of dishwater-coloured fluid, pus exudate or necrotic tissue would be suggestive of diagnosis. If the tissue dissects easily with minimal resistance, the "finger sweep test" is positive.

What are the intraoperative findings in necrotising fasciitis?

Necrotic tissue, fascial oedema, vessel thrombosis, dishwater-coloured fluid and pus.
Minimal resistance required to dissect subcutaneous fascia off deep fascia.

Name 3 risk factors for the development of necrotising fasciitis

- Immunocompromise (e.g. diabetes mellitus, HIV, malignancy, on immunosuppression medications, malnutrition)
- Postsurgery
- Trauma (e.g. IVDU injection sites, burns, lacerations)

What is the prognosis of necrotising fasciitis?

Early diagnosis and prompt debridement of necrotic tissue in necrotising fasciitis improves survival rate. Reconstruction for coverage of soft tissue defect is usually required at a later stage.
Mortality rate had been reported to be between 20-50%. Mortality rates vary according to comorbidities, coexisting infections and duration of time from presentation to surgical debridement.

After wound debridement, the patient recovered with intravenous antibiotics. Skin grafting is required for wound closure. What are the contraindications to skin grafting?

General factors: patient's fitness for surgery
Local wound factors: such as wound vascularity, oxygenation, presence of necrotic tissue or positive growth of microorganisms that might interfere with graft take.

SUMMARY

Necrotising fasciitis is a life threatening condition, which requires a high index of suspicion, early recognition and treatment. Risk factors, which should increase suspicion, include immunocompromise, trauma and post-op patients. Presenting signs and symptoms include intense pain, oedema extending beyond the area of erythema, blisters and palpable crepitus. Diagnosis can be confirmed preoperatively by performing "finger sweep test".

TOP TIPS

➕ Necrotising fasciitis may not always present with pain. Patients can present with haemodynamic instability with nonspecific symptoms. Beware of patient's background risk factors, which may predispose them to developing necrotising fasciitis.

➕ When suspicion of necrotising fasciitis is raised, always escalate the case to seniors promptly, being aware of the severity of the condition, which can eventually be life threatening.

➕ The black-purple tinge of the rash together with a rash that spreads quickly 'in front of your eyes' carry a high index of suspicion.

➕ In cases such as necrotising fasciitis, which require prompt surgical intervention, an understanding of the role of a junior doctor in preparing the patient for surgery is vital. This includes liaising with senior surgeons, anaesthetist, theatre coordinator, patients and their family members.

CLINICAL

3.12 | Right Iliac Fossa Pain

Scenario

You are called to review a 20-year-old female who presented with a 72 hour history of right iliac fossa pain. On approaching the patient, you noticed that she appears to be very pale and much prefers to lie still. Her vital signs are: respiratory rate 25, heart rate 110, temperature 38.8°C, blood pressure 90/60 and SaO2 of 98% on room air.

What is your differential diagnosis?

General surgical causes

- Acute appendicitis
- Meckel's diverticulitis
- Perforated viscous

Gynaecological causes

- Right sided ovarian torsion
- Ectopic pregnancy
- Pelvic inflammatory disease

Urological causes

- Urinary tract infection
- Renal stone

How would you acutely manage this patient?

From the information given, this patient is haemodynamically unstable. Approach the patient in a structured manner.

Airway and Breathing: application of oxtgen and thorough chest examination to look out for any signs of infection in view of pyrexia.
Circulation: Be aware of signs of shock, looking for pallor, cyanosis, decreased capillary refill time and decreased urine output. Fluid resuscitation should be commenced, with strict input and output monitoring. In this case, septic shock due to vasodilation is the most likely cause.
Disability: assess GCS, as reduced alertness indicates cerebral hypoperfusion. Check blood glucose level.
Exposure: thorough abdominal examination and examinations of all systems.

AMPLE history

The need for emergency surgery may be identified, in which case the senior surgeon, emergency theatre coordinator and on call anaesthetist need to be informed.
Keep the patient nil by mouth while awaiting investigations or emergency sur-

CLINICAL

gery.
Sepsis bundle should be commenced, with intravenous antibiotics administered to improve prognosis.

What investigations or tests should be taken or checked to aid your diagnosis?

Baseline bloods: FBC, U&Es, LFTs, CRP, glucose, blood cultures.
ABG (with lactate level).
Urine dip: to rule out urosepsis.
Pregnancy test: positive in ectopic pregnancy.
Erect CXR: free gas under diaphragm in case of perforated viscous.
Ultrasound: abdo/pelvis +/- transvaginal ultrasound.
CT abdomen/pelvis.

What are the specific examination signs that may be positive in acute appendicitis?

Rovsing sign: palpation of left iliac fossa triggers right iliac fossa pain. Suggests peritoneal irritation.
Rebound tenderness
Psoas sign: right iliac fossa pain brought on by extension of right hip or flexion of right hip against resistance.
Obturator sign: right iliac fossa pain brought on by internal rotation or external rotation of flexed right hip.

What are the potential complications of acute appendicitis if left untreated?

Sepsis. In more severe cases, septic shock and multi-organ failure.
Chronic appendicitis.
Periappendicular abcess.
Perforation of appendix.
Death.

Compared to acute cholecystitis, which mostly settles with antibiotics and is managed by planned cholecystectomy at a later stage, why is urgent appedicectomy the mainstay of management for acute appendicitis?

The appendix is supplied by the appendicular branch of the ileocaecal artery, which is an end artery. In acute appendicitis, the appendicular artery can become thrombosed, which results in gangrene and a perforated appendix. To prevent this, acute appendicitis is managed by urgent appendicectomy.
In contrast, the gall bladder is supplied by the cystic artery and right hepatic artery. Hence, if one of the two blood vessels becomes thombosed in acute cholecystitis, the blood supply may not be compromised. Conservative management of acute cholecystitis is usually trialled, with urgent cholecystectomy being considered if the cholecystitis does not settle.

CLINICAL

SUMMARY

Right iliac fossa pain has a broad differential diagnosis covering different specialties. Despite acute appendicitis being an important consideration, gynaecological causes must be considered in a female of childbearing age. Although acute appendicitis is common, it is vital to note that patients can potentially become very unwell, and that resuscitation and emergency appendicectomy is sometimes lifesaving.

It may sometimes be difficult to be certain of a diagnosis preoperatively, in which case discussion with the gynaecology team with an agreement of a gynaecological opinion during a diagnostic laparoscopy procedure may be sensible.

TOP TIPS

➕ A pregnancy test must be performed when a female patient of child bearing age presents with right iliac fossa pain or suprapubic pain.

➕ Be familiar with the anatomy of the appendix, as appendicitis is one of the commonest general surgery pathology and appendicectomy is certainly one of the first surgical procedures that a general surgery SHO will be expected to get involved in.

➕ Be aware of different consent forms, as acute appendicitis can present in people of different ages and it is common to be asked in an interview to discuss usage of different consent forms in different groups of patients.

➕ Consent form 1: Patient agreement for those with capacity to do so.

➕ Consent form 2: Parental agreement for a child or young person.

➕ Consent form 3: Patient/parental agreement to investigation or treatment procedures with no consciousness impairment, i.e. under local anaesthesia.

➕ Consent form 4: Used for adult patients who lack the capacity to consent for themselves. Two senior clinicians are needed to sign this form and it must be a decision made in the patient's best interest, having had a discussion with the patient's next of kin if possible.

3.13 | Loin Pain

Scenario

You are asked to see an 80-year-old lady in A&E. Her only past medical history is hypertension for which she takes amlodipine. She has presented with acute left sided loin pain. She looks unwell, she is clammy and pale and her heart rate is 100bpm.

What is your differential diagnosis?

Ruptured AAA, pyelonephritis, renal colic, diverticulitis

How would you acutely manage this patient?

The patient sounds very unwell so I would ask for help from a senior immediately and would go on to manage this patient using an ABCDE approach. I would measure her respiratory rate and oxygen saturations and give high-flow oxygen through a non-rebreathing mask. I would measure her blood pressure, heart rate and capillary refill and insert two wide-bore cannulae into both antecubital fossae, take blood for testing and cross-match 10 units of blood. If her blood pressure was within normal range I would be cautious about giving IV fluids. I would have the patient catheterised, test the urine and measure her temperature. I would then take a history and examine the patient, focusing on the abdomen/flanks and feeling for a pulsatile expansile mass. If I was concerned that this patient may have a ruptured AAA I would contact surgical/vascular seniors urgently and alert theatres.

How would you differentiate between the different diagnoses?

A patient with a ruptured AAA is likely to describe sudden onset severe abdominal or flank pain. Patients with renal colic tend to describe pain that comes and goes and builds up in severity, and will be unable to lie still. A patient with pyelonephritis or diverticulitis may be unwell from sepsis and have warm peripheries as a result of vasodilation and would likely be pyrexial.

What investigations could aid your diagnosis?

Bloods: FBC, U&Es, LFTs, coagulation screen
Urine dip
ECG
ABG
FAST USS in A&E
CT aortogram

What are the risk factors for AAAs?

- Male sex
- Smoking
- Increasing age
- Family history
- Hypertension
- Hypercholesterolemia
- Marfan syndrome
- Ehlers-Danlos syndrome

What are the indications for operating on patients with known AAAs?

Symptomatic AAAs (back or abdominal pain)
Aneurysm diameter ≥ 5.5cm
Growth of > 0.5cm in 6 months

Would you aggressively give fluids to a patient with a ruptured AAA?

If the patient's blood pressure were within the normal range I would avoid giving IV fluids. The end goal of treatment is to surgically control the source of bleeding but in the meantime it is important to balance the goal of organ perfusion against the risk of excessive bleeding by worsening the rupture by accepting a lower-than-normal blood pressure. This concept is known as 'permissive hypotension'.

What treatment options do you know for treating unruptured AAAs?

Firstly there are lifestyle modifications such as smoking cessation. Medical management includes the use of antihypertensives to reduce the risk of rupture by controlling blood pressure, and statins. Small aneurysms that do not meet the criteria for surgical intervention should be monitored by USS or CT and the frequency of monitoring depends on the diameter of the aneurysm. Surgical options include open surgical repair and endovascular repair.

What is the difference between a true aneurysm and a false aneurysm?

A true aneurysm is a dilation of artery that involves all three layers of artery wall whereas a false aneurysm (or pseudoaneursym) is communication of blood between layers of the artery wall and the arterial lumen without dilatation of all three layers.

What can you tell me about the screening process for AAAs?

In the UK men aged 65 are invited for an USS of their abdomen. Depending on the size of their abdominal aorta they will either be discharged from screening, have their AAA monitored or be referred to a vascular surgeon.

SUMMARY

Abdominal aortic aneurysm is dilation of the abdominal aorta resulting in a diameter over 3cm. 4% of men aged 65 have an AAA and they are associated with factors that cause atherosclerosis. The majority (95%) are infrarenal i.e. start below the origin of the renal arteries. The majority of AAAs are asymptomatic. The risk of rupture and mortality increases with increasing aneurysm diameter. A ruptured AAA is a surgical emergency and it has an 80% mortality rate. Patients with ruptured AAAs typically present with sudden onset severe epigastric/back/loin pain and may have a history of collapse. They will show signs of shock. If the patient is stable a CT aortogram can be performed to confirm the diagnosis but this shouldn't delay transfer to theatre if the patient is haemodynamically unstable.

TOP TIPS

 You may not always feel a 'pulsatile, expansile abdominal mass' in a patient with a ruptured AAA, due to pain and abdominal wall rigidity

 Don't forget how important escalation is when a patient presents in this way – you will need many experienced hands and minds

CLINICAL

3.14 Acute Leg Pain

Scenario

An overweight 51-year-old gentleman with a background of ischaemic heart disease and type two diabetes presents to A&E with a sudden onset of severe pain in his right leg below the knee

What is your differential diagnosis?

Acutely ischaemic limb (embolic or acute-on-chronic occlusion)
Deep vein thrombosis
Fracture or musculoskeletal injury
Compartment syndrome
Gout

How would you acutely manage this gentleman?

The gentleman should be assessed and resuscitated using an ABCDE approach to identify life-threatening abnormal parameters.
If the gentleman is stable a full history and examination should be performed to elicit the cause of the leg pain. Given the patient's age, history of ischaemic heart disease and diabetes and the sudden onset of the pain the most important condition to identify is an acutely ischaemic limb.

Do not delay simply examining and comparing both lower limbs for peripheral pulses, warmth, colour, altered sensation and muscle power. Document peripheral pulses using a standardised diagram in the notes. Given this gentleman's pain is below his knee an occlusion in the common femoral, superficial femoral or popliteal arteries should be considered and femoral, popliteal, posterior tibial and dorsalis pedis pulses should be recorded.

If pulses are weak or absent a hand-held doppler should be used to assess the arterial waveform and perform ABPIs. Contact the vascular team early and keep the patient starved. Depending on access to scans arterial duplex or CT angiogram should be sought.
Treatment should not be delayed and the limb should be reperfused as quickly as possible:
Immediate: oxygen and IVI fluids, analgesia and heparinise, treat underlying cardiac conditions
Thrombosis in-situ: thrombolysis, angioplasty, bypass surgery
Embolic: embolectomy, thrombolysis
Amputation if irreversible

What key questions in your history might point towards a cause of vascular origin?

Time frame of onset of symptoms (acute without trauma suggests a vascular origin)

Previous history of claudication pain e.g. does s similar pain come on after walking a set distance (claudication distance)
Arteriopath medical history (cardiac history, anticoagulation or diabetes)
Symptoms: 6 P's- pain, pallor, pulseless, perishing cold, paraesthesia, paralysis

What investigations would aid your diagnosis?

Bloods tests: FBC, U&Es, clotting screen
ABPIs
Arterial duplex
CT angiogram

What are the three components of a normal doppler waveform?

* Multiphasic
* Pulsatile
* Regular amplitude

What are the causes of acute limb ischaemia?

Acute Thrombosis In-Situ (60%)
Acute occlusion in a vessel with pre-existing atherosclerosis
Risk factors: dehydration, malignancy, hypotension, prothrombotic disorders
Emboli (30-40%)
Cardiac cause (80%): AF, MI, prosthetic/damaged heart valves
Also from aneurysm, tumour, foreign body
Other causes
Trauma, peripheral aneurysm (popliteal), dissecting aneurysm

How do would differentiate between embolism and thrombosis as a cause?

In chronic disease collateral vessles have time to form to try to bypss the blockage making the onset of symptoms slower.

Clinical features	Embolus	Thrombosis
Severity	Complete (no collaterals)	Incomplete (collaterals)
Onset	Seconds/ Minutes	Hours/days
Multiple sites	Up to 15%	Rare
Embolic source	Present	Absent
Previous claudication	Absent	Present
Palpation of artery	Soft, tender	Hard, calcified
Bruits	Absent	Present
Contralateral leg pulses	Present	Absent

CLINICAL

How do the results of ABPIs relate to diagnosis?

- Normal: >0.7
- Intermittent: 0.7-0.9
- Rest pain: 0.5
- Critical ischaemia: <0.3

What are the complications of an ischaemic limb?

Loss of limb (40%): irreversible tissue damage at 6hrs
Death (20%)
Reperfusion syndrome: free radical release causing compartment syndrome and chronic pain
Complications from thrombolysis: CVE, retroperitoneal bleed

SUMMARY

Acute limb ischaemia is caused by a sudden decrease in the blood flow to a limb, which results in a threat to the viability of the limb. Systemic acid base and electrolyte disturbances can occur due to the hypoperfusion, which in turn can impair renal and cardiopulmonary function. Highly toxic free radicals can be released when the limb is reperfused which can lead to compartment syndrome and chronic pain. The classical description of patients with acute limb ischemia is represented by the "six Ps": pain, pallor, paralysis, pulseless, paraesthesia, and perishing cold. The duration of symptoms is of upmost importance in planning treatment and urgency can make the difference between complete recovery, amputation and death.

TOP TIPS

➕ A high index of suspicion should be had when assessing arteriopaths who present with sudden onset pain. Vascular surgeons should be contacted early, imaging organised and IV heparin given within an hour of a presumed acutely ischaemic limb as time can save limbs.

➕ Distinguishing between acute ischaemia and chronic occlusive disease is important in deciding upon management, knowledge of differentiating symptoms is important.

➕ Knowledge of the pathophysiology of reperfusion syndrome and how to minimise the effects of it are key to reducing the morbidity and mortality of an ischaemic vessel.

CLINICAL

3.15 | Stab Wound

Scenario

You are called to ED to assess a 20-year-old man who was stabbed in the back during a fight. He is talking to you but appears slightly confused. He complains of chest pain and breathlessness. The wound on the back is between the shoulder blades; it is not actively bleeding and appears clean. The patient is tachycardic and tachypnoeic.

What is your differential diagnosis?

- Haemothorax
- Pneumothorax *(tension or open)*
- Cardiac tamponade
- Thoracic aorta or great vessels dissection/injury
- Flail chest with lung contusion

How would you acutely manage this patient?

The patient has sustained a major trauma and should be managed following an ABCDE approach using ATLS protocols identifying and treating life-threatening conditions.

Airway and C-Spine: triple C-spine immobilisation should be established and maintained until cervical spine integrity is confirmed. The airway should be checked using the 'look, listen and feel' approach, with immediate treatment if there is airway compromise. Neck extension and chin lift are impossible with C-spine immobilisation. Simple manoeuvres and adjuncts should be tried first and anaesthetic help sought early if the need to advanced airway management is anticipated.

Breathing: breathing and ventilation should be assessed using the 'look, listen and feel' technique. The application of 15L oxygen via a non-rebreathe mask is standard in any trauma patient, irrespective of the presence of COPD. Palpate the trachea (is it central?) and check to see if the neck veins are distended. Percuss the chest to check if it is resonant (normal), tympanic (suggestive pneumothorax) or dull (suggestive of haemothorax). Inspect the chest to look for an open pneumothorax ('sucking chest wound') or evidence of flail chest (segment of the chest wall moving paradoxically with respiration). Any of those conditions would need to be managed during the primary survey.

Circulation: the next step is to assess circulation with haemorrhage control. Obtain IV access with two large-bore cannulas (at least 16G) and draw blood for baseline tests (see below), including G&S plus/minus cross-match according to the suspicion of acute bleeding. Fluid resuscitation with warmed crystalloid solution (initial bolus 30 ml/kg) should be started whilst further assessment is undertaken. Patients with known heart failure should have the initial bolus reduced to 10 ml/kg. Once monitoring is available, fluid resuscitation should be

CLINICAL

titrated to patient response. Bleeding should always be considered the cause of circulatory dysfunction in the trauma patient, until proven otherwise. Look for hidden sources of bleeding – 'on the floor and four more (abdomen/pelvis, retroperitoneum, long bones and chest). Prompt haemorrhage control is mandatory with either external compression or surgery.

Disability: rapid assessment of neurologic dysfunction is performed by examining the pupils and using the GCS system. Blood glucose should also be assessed and corrected accordingly. Appropriate analgesia should be administered to ensure the patient is comfortable (IV morphine is the preferred therapy in the trauma setting).

Exposure: the initial survey is completed by exposure and examination of the patient (preserving dignity and minimising thermal losses). Log roll can be performed at this stage if not yet done.

Adjuncts to the primary survey include ABG, nasogastric tube, urinary catheter, ECG, chest, C-spine and pelvis radiographs, and FAST (Focused Assessment with Sonography in Trauma).

Once the primary survey is completed, the next steps are AMPLE story and secondary survey, which includes full examination to diagnose lesions that were initially missed in the primary survey.

What investigation would aid your diagnosis?

Blood tests: FBC; U&Es; LFTs; amylase; clotting and G&S (remember β-hCG if female)

ABG/VBG: acid-basic status, lactate; immediate Hb and electrolytes; $pO2$ and $pCO2$

Chest, C-spine and pelvic XR: to investigate for pneumothorax/rib fracture; C-spine fracture; pelvic fracture (?bleeding ?urethral injury)

FAST: intra-abdominal fluid (means blood until proven otherwise)

Full trauma series CT scan: thorax, abdomen, pelvis; head and neck if appropriate

How would you clinically distinguish between a tension pneumothorax and a massive haemothorax?

Both conditions are life-threatening as they affect breathing and ventilation as well as circulation (increased intra-thoracic pressure prevents venous return). Tension pneumothorax is characterised by distended neck veins, ipsilateral tympanic hemi-thorax, tracheal deviation towards the contralateral side and silent hemi-thorax (absent breathing sounds). A massive haemothorax also presents with tracheal deviation towards the contralateral side and ipsilateral silent hemi-thorax, but neck veins are collapsed (due to hypovolaemia) and there is dullness to percussion on the ipsilateral side.

What is the definition of massive haemothorax? And how you manage it?

Massive haemothorax is characterised by immediate drainage of more than 1500 ml of blood on insertion of chest drain or more than 200 ml/hr for 2 hours. In addition to resuscitation (including RBC transfusion), immediate management includes insertion of a chest drain, followed by surgical exploration to control the haemorrhagic source.

The observations for this patient are RR 30, HR 120 and BP 90/70. Which stage of haemorrhagic shock is the patient? Why? What can you anticipate?

The patient is in stage III of haemorrhagic shock because he is tachycardic and hypotensive, despite a decreased pulse pressure. Resuscitation will need transfusion of RBC and blood products on top of crystalloids.

	I	II	III	IV
Blood loss (mL)	<750	750-1500	1500-2000	>2000
Blood loss (%blood volume)	<15	15-30	30-40	>40
Pulse (per minute)	<100	100-120	120-140	>140
Blood pressure (mmHg)	Normal	Normal	Decreased	Decreased
Pulse pressure (mmHg)	Normal or increased	Decreased	Decreased	Decreased
RR (per minute)	14-20	20-30	30-40	>35
Urine output (mL/h)	>30	20-30	5-15	Negligible
Mental status	Slightly anxious	Mildly anxious	Anxious, confused	Lethargic

After 1.5 L of Hartmann's, the patient has BP 110/80 and HR 110. However, as IV fluids are slowed down, he rapidly deteriorates again. How would you classify his response? What do you do?

The patient needs to be re-assessed using the ABCDE approach, managing abnormalities as they are encountered. The patient had a transient response to crystalloids but haemodynamic instability recurred. Therefore, he needs RBC and blood product transfusion and prompt exploration and haemorrhage control, as he seems to be actively bleeding.

The CT scan shows active extravasation of contrast from the posterior intercostal arteries. Whilst the patient is being prepared to go to theatre, what BP would you aim for?

Permissive hypotension should govern resuscitation when the patient is actively bleeding. The aim is to ensure vital organs are adequately perfused whilst the BP is kept low to minimise bleeding. A systolic BP of 90 mmHg is generally used as target but it should be adjusted on an individual basis.

Where do you insert a chest drain?

A chest drain should be inserted in the fifth intercostal space, just anterior to the

CLINICAL

middle axillary line. This coincides with the 'triangle of safety', which is bounded by the lateral border of pectoralis major anteriorly, the anterior border of latissimus dorsi posteriorly and the 5th intercostal space inferiorly (a line passing horizontally through the nipple). The apex is the axilla. For a haemothorax the drain is directed downwards, whilst for a pneumothorax it is directed upwards. The drain should be connected to a closed system with/without suction. Correct position is suggested by bubbling and swinging but it should be confirmed with chest radiograph.

SUMMARY

Penetrating chest trauma is not uncommon and can cause life-threatening haemorrhage in cases when the aorta and great vessels are affected. Any injury located in between the scapulae mandates exclusion of tamponade. Other injuries to look for and manage in the primary survey include tension or open pneumothorax, massive haemothorax and flail chest with lung contusion. Shock in the context of trauma is hypovolaemic and more specifically haemorrhagic until proven otherwise. According to clinical assessment, patients can be categorised into one of 4 stages of shock, which can help making treatment decisions. The response to initial resuscitation guides further management – transient responders and non-responders require more aggressive resuscitation with blood products and likely surgical intervention to control haemorrhage.

TOP TIPS

➕ Tension pneumothorax is a clinical diagnosis *(never ask for a chest radiograph!)*, which requires immediate needle decompression *(large-bore cannula inserted in the 2nd intercostal space, midclavicular line)* followed by a chest drain *(the needle thoracostomy only buys you about 20 minutes)*

➕ Remember the 'lethal triad in trauma' – acidosis, coagulopathy and hypothermia

➕ If there is any change in the patient's condition, always re-assess following the ABCDE approach *(even if the interviewers try to point you in the direction of a 'C' problem)*

➕ If you don't feel comfortable managing the airway or inserting a chest drain on your own, say that you would ask for help – you will get Brownie points for showing that you have self-awareness and prioritise patient's safety instead of risking doing something for which you are not thoroughly competent

3.16 | Acute Groin Pain

> ## Scenario
>
> An 80-year-old lady presents with abdominal pain, distension and vomiting. She has had absolute constipation for 48 hours. She is dehydrated and tachycardic. The abdomen is distended but soft and there is tenderness in the left groin on palpation with a small hard mass present.

What is your differential diagnosis?

Small bowel obstruction secondary to a (incarcerated) femoral hernia or (incarcerated) inguinal hernia
Lymphadenopathy
Saphenous varix
Lipoma
Femoral aneurysm
Psoas abscess
AAA

How would you acutely manage this patient?

The patient should be stabilised following an ABCDE approach.

Airway: the airway should be checked using the 'look, listen and feel' approach, with immediate treatment if there is airway compromise. Simple manoeuvres and adjuncts should be tried first and anaesthetic help sought early if the need to advanced airway management is anticipated.

Breathing: provided that the airway is patent, breathing should be assessed using also the 'look, listen and feel' technique. The application of 15L oxygen via a non-rebreathe mask is standard in any acutely unwell patient, irrespective of the presence of COPD.

Circulation: the next step is to assess circulation and obtain IV access with two large-bore cannulas (at least 16G) and draw blood for baseline tests (see below), including G&S plus/minus cross-match according to the suspicion of acute bleeding. Fluid resuscitation with warmed crystalloid solution (initial bolus 10 ml/kg if normal haemodynamic parameters or 30 ml/kg if hypotension) should be started whilst further assessment is undertaken. Patients with known heart failure should have the initial bolus reduced to 5 ml/kg). Hypovolaemia should always be considered the cause of circulatory dysfunction in the surgical patient, until proven otherwise. Once monitoring is available, fluid resuscitation should be titrated to patient response.

The patient should be catheterised to monitor fluid balance and appropriate analgesia should be administered to ensure the patient is comfortable.

Disability: rapid assessment of neurologic dysfunction is performed by examining the pupils and using the AVPU system (alert, responds to voice, responds to pain, unresponsive).

Exposure: the initial assessment is completed by exposure and examination of the patient (preserving dignity and minimising thermal losses). Once the patient is stable, the focus can shift to identifying the underlying condition and its aetiology in order to put in place an adequate management plan.

What investigation would aid your diagnosis?

Blood tests: FBC (?infection, anaemia); U&Es (?dehydration, AKI, electrolyte disturbances, baseline renal function anticipating need for CT scan); CRP (?infection/inflammation); clotting (?pre-op/bleeding) and G&S (?pre-op/bleeding)

ABG/VBG: acid-basic status, lactate; immediate Hb and electrolytes (anaerobic metabolism is associated with shock; electrolyte disturbances and anaemia may require immediate correction); ABG additionally provides pO2 if there are concerns about airway and/or breathing

Chest XR: to investigate for free air under the diaphragm and as pre-op requirement

Abdominal XR: of doubtful use when CT scan is easily available; may show abnormal distribution of bowel gas, dilated bowel loops. The definitive imaging is CT scan to show the underlying aetiology.

CT scan abdomen and pelvis with IV contrast: to investigate cause for bowel obstruction: hernia, carcinoma, volvulus, etc. It will also rule out an AAA!

Inguinal USS: to investigate for inguinal/femoral hernias, vascular abnormalities, lymphadenopathy. CT scan is usually the first choice as it provides more information than USS, which is an alternative if CT scan is not readily available.

The AXR shows dilated small bowel loops. What is your working diagnosis and what are the main causes?

Bowel obstruction (SBO/LBO)
SBO: adhesions (post-operative), incarcerated hernias
LBO: carcinoma, volvulus

How do you differentiate between SB and LB loops on the plain abdominal film?

SBO: predominantly central, valvulae conniventes (aka Kerckring folds or plicae circulares) cross the entire lumen, diameter <3 cm
LBO: follow the abdominal contour (peripheral), haustrations only cross one-third of the lumen on each side, diameter <6 cm (diameter <9 cm for caecum)

What are the most common hernias? And what hernia would you expect in this old lady?

Inguinal hernias (mostly direct). Indirect hernias are more common in children. Remember that femoral hernias typically present in old females but even in this population, inguinal hernias are more frequent than femoral hernias.

The CT scan confirmed the presence of a femoral hernia. Can you described the anatomical relations of the hernia sac? And what is usually contained within it?

A femoral hernia is an abnormal protrusion of a peritoneum-lined sac through

CLINICAL

the femoral canal, which lies medially to the femoral sheath beneath the inguinal ligament and laterally to the lacunar ligament and pubis. The femoral canal usually contains fat and the lymph node of Cloquet. Laterally to the femoral canal lies the femoral sheath, which encloses the femoral artery and vein from lateral to medial. The femoral nerve lies laterally to the femoral artery. The great saphenous vein pierces the cribiform fascia to drain into the femoral vein about 2 cm laterally and inferiorly to the pubic tubercle. All these important structures in the vicinity of the femoral hernia are not only sources of differential diagnosis but also potentially damaged during hernia repair.

SUMMARY

Incarcerated hernias are a common cause of small bowel obstruction, only second to post-operative adhesions. Inguinal hernias are more frequent than femoral hernias and the latter typically presents in elderly female patients. Acute management involves haemodynamic stabilisation followed by urinary catheterisation to accurately measure fluid balance and hence guide fluid resuscitation. NG tube insertion is usual required to prevent vomiting and aspiration. CT scan with contrast (abdomen and pelvis) is the imaging of choice to identify the aetiology, delineate the transition point and rule out other life-threatening conditions (e.g. AAA) or undiagnosed malignancy (particularly in the elderly). Surgical repair is mandatory for femoral hernias due to the high risk of incarceration and/or strangulation.

TOP TIPS

➕ Don't forget about AAAs presenting as left loin/groin pain *(the examiners won't forgive you for missing that!)*

➕ Femoral hernias are more common in elderly females but inguinal hernias remain the most frequent type of hernias even in that population *(femora hernias are rare!)*

➕ Remember that 'drip and suck' remains the basic management of bowel obstruction – that together with requesting CT scan and routine blood tests is what will be expected from a core surgical trainee.

CLINICAL

3.17 | Acute Epigastric Pain

Scenario

A 42-year-old woman presents with a 12-hour history of nausea, vomiting and epigastric pain, which radiates to her back. Her abdomen is tender in the epigastrium. She is hypotensive and tachycardic. She is obese but otherwise healthy. There is no previous history of any abdominal pain. She denies drinking and smoking and she lives with her husband and four children.

What is your differential diagnosis?

Pancreatitis
AAA
Cholecystitis
Bowel obstruction/perforation
Peptic ulceration
Diabetic ketoacidosis

How would you initially manage this patient?

The patient should be stabilised following an ABCDE approach.

Airway: The airway should be checked using the 'look, listen and feel' approach, with immediate treatment if there is airway compromise. Simple manoeuvres and adjuncts should be tried first and anaesthetic help sought early if the need to advanced airway management is anticipated.

Breathing: Breathing should be assessed using also the 'look, listen and feel' technique. The application of 15L oxygen via a non-rebreathe mask is standard in any acutely unwell patient, irrespective of the presence of COPD.

Circulation: Obtain IV access with two large-bore cannulas (at least 16G) and draw blood for baseline tests (see below), including G&S plus/minus crossmatch according to the suspicion of acute bleeding. Fluid resuscitation with warmed crystalloid solution (initial bolus 10 ml/kg if normal haemodynamic parameters or 30 ml/kg if hypotension) should be started whilst further assessment is undertaken. Patients with known heart failure should have the initial bolus reduced to 5 ml/kg). Hypovolaemia should always be considered the cause of circulatory dysfunction in the surgical patient, until proven otherwise. Once monitoring is available, fluid resuscitation should be titrated to patient response. The patient should be catheterised to monitor fluid balance and appropriate analgesia should be administered to ensure the patient is comfortable.

Disability: Rapid assessment of neurologic dysfunction is performed by examining the pupils and using the AVPU system (alert, responds to voice, responds to pain, unresponsive).

Exposure: The initial assessment is completed by exposure and examination of the patient (preserving dignity and minimising thermal losses).

Once the patient is stable, the focus can shift to identifying the underlying condition and its aetiology in order to put in place an adequate management plan.

What investigations would you order?

Blood tests: FBC (?infection/inflammation, anaemia); U&Es (?dehydration, AKI, electrolyte disturbances); LFTs (?cholestasis, liver disease); amylase/lipase (?pancreatitis); CRP (?infection/inflammation); LDH (?pancreatitis); glucose; clotting (?bleeding/liver dysfunction) and G&S

ABG/VBG: acid-basic status, lactate; immediate Hb and electrolytes (anaerobic metabolism is associated with shock; electrolyte disturbances and anaemia may require immediate correction); ABG additionally provides pO2 and pCO2 if there are concerns about airway and/or breathing (?ARDS, scoring)

Chest XR: to investigate for free air under the diaphragm

Abdominal USS: to investigate for gallstones and exclude AAA

The amylase comes back as 1000 U/L. What is your diagnosis? Can you name any other causes?

Acute pancreatitis

The most common likely cause is gallstones because this patient fits with the typical picture 'forty, fat, female and fertile'. There is also no history of alcohol excess, which is the second most common aetiology. The mnemonic **I GET SMASHED** can help you remember other less frequent causes:

I – Idiopathic
G – Gallstones (60%)
E – Ethanol (30%)
T – Trauma
S – Steroids
M – Mumps
A – Autoimmune (e.g. SLE)
S – Scorpion bites (rare!)
H – Hypercalcaemia, hypothermia, hyperlipidaemia
E – ERCP
D – Drugs (e.g. azathioprine, NSAIDs, thiazides, isoniazid)

What scoring systems do you know to classify the severity of acute pancreatitis?

APACHE II, Ranson, BISAP and Glasgow. The modified Glasgow (Imrie) score is the most widely used to assess prognostic severity.

Would you request a CT scan for this patient?

CT scan should not be requested in the first 48-72h after symptom onset because inflammatory changes are often not radiographically present until after this time. It is seldom indicated for patients with mild pancreatitis unless a pancreatic carcinoma is suspected (usually in elderly patients). It is always indicated in patients with severe acute pancreatitis and is the imaging study of choice for assessing complications. Abdominal CT scan can also provide prognostic information based on radiologic severity criteria, which can help stratify the risk of necrosis and subsequent infection.

CLINICAL

What are some of the complications of acute pancreatitis?

Pancreatic pseudocyst, pancreatic necrosis (sterile or infected), haemorrhage (intra- or retroperitoneal), chronic pancreatitis, ARDS, death

SUMMARY

The cardinal symptoms of acute pancreatitis is abdominal pain, which is often located in the upper abdomen, usually in the epigastric region, but it may be perceived more on the left or right side, depending on which portion of the pancreas is involved. The pain radiates directly through the abdomen to the back and is relieved by sitting forward. Nausea and vomiting are often present along with accompanying anorexia. Suspicions should be raised in patients with a history of gallstones, alcohol excess, recent ERCP or hypertriglyceridemia. On examination, patients can be tender with guarding on the epigastrium. Cullen's sign (periumbilical bruising) and Grey-Turner's sign (bilateral flank bruising indicating pancreatic necrosis with retroperitoneal bleeding) are classical but seldom encountered. Immediate management should focus on fluid resuscitation due to significant intracompartmental fluid shifts, analgesia and anti-emesis. Scoring on admission and in 48h, generally using the Glasgow scoring system, is crucial for prognosis and decision making regarding treatment and escalation to ITU for more advanced monitoring and support in cases of severe pancreatitis. Treatment is mainly supportive and nutrition, either through enteral or parenteral route, should not be overlooked, Complications can be local or systemic. Local complications include pseudocyst formation or pancreatic necrosis (sterile or infected), which tend to occur in 10-12 days of the acute event; systemic complications can manifest as SIRS with multi-organ failure and even death – the lung and kidney are frequently affected with ARDS and AKI, respectively.

TOP TIPS

➕ Do not forget about the history of alcohol abuse. Not only is this a cause of pancreatitis but also needs addressing in itself – prevent Wernicke's encephalopathy and alcohol withdrawal

➕ Abdominal USS should be obtained early to confirm aetiology and assess need for intervention *(ERCP if stones obstructing CBD)*

➕ ITU support is mandatory for severe pancreatitis as there is a significant risk of complications, which require organ support and/or replacement *(ARDS, severe AKI...)*

➕ Cholecystectomy is the definitive treatment for gallstone pancreatitis. ERCP with sphincterotomy is the alternative for patients considered unfit for surgery

3.18 | Testicular Swelling

Scenario

You are asked to see a 21-year-old male patient in A&E who has presented with a right sided swollen testicle. He is otherwise fit and well and is not yet sexually active.

What is your differential diagnosis?

Testicular torsion
Epididymo-orchitis/orchitis
Varicocele, hydrocele, haematocele
Testicular tumour
Hernia
Epididymal cyst
Mumps

Testicular torsion is an emergency and you should rule this out in the first instance. Epididymo-orchitis is a very common presentation.

How would you acutely manage this patient?

 "I would manage this patient by following an ABCDE approach according to ATLS principles. I don't expect him to have any issues with his airway or breathing but I would like to know his basic observations including oxygen saturations, respiratory rate, heart rate, blood pressure, capillary refill and his temperature. As part of my initial assessment/management of circulation I would get IV access and take bloods and consider IV fluids in the form of a fluid challenge. I would take a full history and examine the patient's abdomen and external genitalia. If there was any evidence of tosion or compromise of the testicle I would inform the surgical/urological registrar immediately, keep the patient starved and optimise him for theatre. If he appeared stable and there was no clear evidence of compromise I would proceed to order appropriate investigations."

What investigations would aid your diagnosis?

FBC, U&Es, LFTS, CRP, coagulation, G&S
Urinalysis
Testicular USS
Transillumination of scrotum
STI test

The patient is haemodynamically stable and apyrexial. His blood tests and urine dip are unremarkable. On examination of his external genitalia you find a non-tender, irregular, firm lump fixed to the right testis, which you can get above.

What do you think is the most likely diagnosis?

Testicular cancer, which would most likely be a teratoma in this patient given his age.

What are the different types of testicular cancer?

The most common types are seminoma and teratoma (non-seminomatous germ cell tumours). Other types of non-seminomatous germ cell tumours include choriocarcinoma and yolk sac tumours. A rare type of testicular cancer is lymphoma.

How would the clinical picture differ if this patient had testicular torsion?

The patient is likely to have presented with sudden onset severe pain which may be associated with nausea, vomiting and abdominal pain. On examination the testis is globally tender, enlarged, high-riding in the scrotum and may have a transverse axis. There may also be absence of the cremasteric reflex on the affected side.

What would you do next to manage the patient with suspected testicular cancer?

The patient needs an urgent two-week wait referral to urology. In the meantime I would ensure tumour markers (AFP, β-HCG, LDH) have been sent off. He will ultimately need a CT chest and abdomen and an orchidectomy carried out as soon as possible. Sperm storage should be considered.

Do you know any risk factors for testicular cancer?
- Family history
- Down syndrome
- Klinefelter syndrome
- Cryptorchidism

What surgical approach is used when performing an orchidectomy for testicular cancer and why?

An inguinal approach should be performed as opposed to a scrotal approach.

This is so that the spermatic cord can be cross-clamped prior to mobilising the testis to prevent dissemination of cancer cells along lymphatics, as well as allowing for ligation of the testicular lymphatics as high as possible as they pass in the spermatic cord and through the internal inguinal ring to remove any cancer cells which may have metastasized along the cord. It also prevents dissemination of tumour cells into the lymphatics that drain the scrotal skin that could

CLINICAL

occur if a scrotal approach were used (the testes drain into para-aortic lymph nodes whereas inguinal nodes drain the scrotal skin).

What is the prognosis for testicular cancer?

Typically good prognosis for cancer confined to the testis (>95%). Cure rate of 80% in metastatic cancer.

SUMMARY

Testicular cancer is the commonest malignancy in men between the ages of 18 and 40. The incidence of seminomas is higher in men between the age of 30-40 and the incidence of teratomas is higher in men between the age of 20-30. Patients typically present with a painless testicular mass. Orchidectomy is the mainstay of treatment with additional radiotherapy and chemotherapy depending on type of tumour and stage.

TOP TIPS

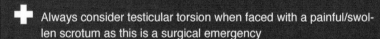 Always consider testicular torsion when faced with a painful/swollen scrotum as this is a surgical emergency

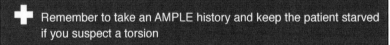 Remember to take an AMPLE history and keep the patient starved if you suspect a torsion

CLINICAL

3.19 | Hip Injury

Scenario

A 45-year-old man is admitted after falling heavily from his mountain bike. He is an engineer, has no past medical history, is a non-smoker and is NV intact with a closed injury to his right hip. A radiograph reveals an intracapsular fractured neck of femur.

How would you acutely manage this patient?

This gentleman should be resuscitated using ATLS protocols to ensure that he is stable and no injuries have been missed. An ABCDE approach should be followed, this is a high energy trauma and other injuries are likely.

Provided the patient is stable and primary and secondary surveys reveal only the intracapsular fracture management may then focus on this.

An intracapsular fracture in a young adult (<65 years) requires prompt, anatomical reduction to preserve blood supply to the femoral head.

What investigations would you request?

Investigations in this case are to optimise the patient for theatre rather than aid diagnosis as a radiograph has already confirmed the diagnosis.
FBC, U&Es, LFTs, CRP, coagulation, G&S

What is the blood supply to the femoral head and why is it important in this case?

The main supply to the femoral head is from the trochanteric anastomosis formed by the medial and lateral circumflex arteries and superior gluteal artery. There is a small supply from the artery of ligamentum teres (a branch of the obturator artery) and a small supply from vessels running in the medullary canal. In a young adult (<65) the femoral head should be preserved if possible as a hip replacement will likely need a revision in later life.

What is the difference between the above fracture in a 45-year-old and an 85-year-old?

For an elderly patient, the goals are to restore mobility with weight-bearing as tolerated and to minimize complications seen with prolonged bed rest. A hemiarthroplasty or total hip replacement often accomplishes these goals best.
For a physiologically young and active adult, the goals are to preserve the femoral head, avoid osteonecrosis and achieve union. Avoiding an arthroplasty is the goal. It is generally agreed that anatomic reduction and stable internal fixation (cannulated screws or DHS) performed by an experienced surgeon are more important than operating as soon as possible (the old guidance of 'within 6-hours').

In practical terms how quickly would you take this gentleman to theatre?

Timing of surgery is controversial and it is generally agreed that a stable, anatomical reduction performed by an experience surgeon is more desirable than a rushed, non-anatomic result.

In practical terms it is important to find out when the injury took place and what time the patient arrived in the hospital. If it is day time fixing the hip on a consultant list is desirable. If it is out of hours a preferred option may be to delay until the following morning but this should be discussed with the consultant on call.

How would you manage this gentleman post-operatively?

Unlike hip fractures in the elderly which aim to get patients fully weight-bearing on day one to avoid complications secondary to immobility young adults should be mobilise NWB/PWB on crutches for 6 weeks to facilitate fracture healing.

How many hip fractures are there approximately in the UK each year and what is their morbidity and mortality?

Over 70,000 hip fractures occur annually in the UK. The total cost of care is over £2 billion with 10% mortality at 30 days and up to 30% mortality at one year.

What guidelines do you know for managing intracapsular hip fractures in the elderly popilation? Can you summarise the key points?

NICE and the British Orthopaedic Association (BOA) have produced a set of guidelines aimed at managing all hip fractures in the elderly. For intracapsular fractures the key managment points include:

- Operate on patients with the aim to allow them to fully weight bear *(without restriction)* in the immediate postoperative period
- Perform replacement arthroplasty in patients with a displaced intracapsular fracture
- Offer total hip replacements to patients with a displaced intracapsular fracture who:
  - were able to walk independently and
  - are not cognitively impaired and
  - are medically fit for anaesthesia and the procedure
- Use a proven femoral stem design rather than an Austin Moore or Thompson stems for arthroplasties
- Use cemented implants in patients undergoing surgery with arthroplasty
- Consider an anterolateral approach in favour of a posterior approach when inserting a hemiarthroplasty
- Review by an orthogeriatric medical team

SUMMARY

Hip fractures are very common with over 70,000 occurring annually in the UK. Patients tend to be elderly with osteoporosis and significant comorbidities meaning that any period of immobility increases their risk or infection, thrombosis and death. Operating and mobilising patients within 48 hours has been shown to dramatically reduce both morbidity and mortality and NICE and the BOA have published guidelines to optimise the care of patients with hip fractures. For intracapsular fractures (when femoral head blood supply is compromised) a cemented hemiartroplasty should be used in patients with limited mobility and a total hip replacement for patients who walk unrestricted. A dynamic hip screw should be used for pertrochnateric extracapsular fractures and an intramedually nail should be used for patients with subtrochanteric and reverse obliquity fractures.

In the younger age group with non-osteoporotic bone treatment should focus on timely restoration of femoral head blood supply to avoid avascular necorosis and the need for an early hip replacement.

TOP TIPS

➕ Read the BOA standards for trauma before your interview these cover hip fractures, open fractures, pelvic and spinal injuries and nerve injuries www.boa.ac.uk

➕ Elderly hip fracture patients often have significant comorbidities and may be on anticoagulants, have a pacemaker, require fluid resuscitation or be high risk for theatre. Make sure you deal with each of these in turn and ensure they are optimised for theatre and reviewed by the orthogeriatric team both before and after their operation.

➕ In non-osteoporotic patients preservation of the femoral head using cannulated screws or a DHS will avoid the necessity of a hip replacement and subsequent revision *(THRs typically last 15-20 years before loosening).*

3.20 | Paediatric Trauma

> **Scenario**
>
> You are the trauma and orthopaedic SHO on nights and receive a trauma call for a 7-year-old girl who has been hit by a car. She is alert and stable but is holding her right arm whilst lying on a trolley and looks in pain and very upset. The ED consultant thinks she has a fracture to her forearm.

What is your differential diagnosis?

Forearm fracture
Supracondylar fracture
Consider any other concomitant injury given nature of trauma
Consider head injury
Consider non-accidental injury

How would you acutely manage this patient?

A full ATLS primary survey should be undertaken as the mechanism of injury is high energy. An ABCDE approach should be adopted to ensure that the patient is haemodynamically stable prior to any further assessment. Given that this is a child liaising with the on-call paediatric team is sensible. The child will likely be scared and it is important to take this into account.

Fluid resuscitation should be with adjusted volumes and doses for children as should analgesia.

Commence the secondary survey obtaining a more detailed history and mechanism of injury and proceed to examine "head to toe". Neurovascular status of any injury you might find with suspicion of fracture or possible neurovascular damage must be assessed and documented.

Following secondary survey you find a deformity of the right forearm with bruising, tenderness and reduced range of movement likely due to a fracture. You also notice that the child refuses to move her left leg and there is a large haematoma over the anterior aspect of the thigh.

What investigations would aid your diagnosis?

AP and lateral radiographs of right forearm including the joint above and below the injury (elbow and wrist)
Radiographs of left femur including joint above and below (hip and knee) AP and lateral films.

Given that the child is aged 7 how would you assess neurovascular status of the left arm in practical terms?

In children it can be difficult to accurately perform a neurological exam especially if they are distressed. Building rapport and getting them to copy your movements is key to assessing the three peripheral nerves of the upper limb.

Median nerve: assess the anterior interosseous branch of the median nerve (AIN) by asking her to make an 'ok' sign testing flexor policis longus (FPL) and flexor digitorum profundus (FDP) and test sensation over the volar aspect of the index finger.

Ulna nerve: function is assessed by asking her to cross her middle finger over her index finger (testing intrinsic muscles of hand) and sensation over the little finger

Radial nerve: function is assessed by asking her to extend her wrist or metacarpophalangeal joints (MCPJs) and testing sensation over the dorsal 1st webspace.

Check CRT: at the hand and feel for a radial pulse and inspect the colour of the hand compared with the opposite side.

The child is stable and radiographs reveal mid-shaft fractures to her left radius and ulna and a spiral fracture of her left femur. How would you manage her now?

Although stable she is a polytrauma and will likely need timely surgical intervention.

She should be given appropriate analgesia and the fractures should be splinted using an above-elbow backslab for the forearm fractures and a Thomas splint or skin traction for the femoral fracture. Depending on time of day and theatre availability you should keep her starved, inform the orthopaedic registrar and mark and consent her using a consent form 2 after discussion with her legal guardian.

Given her age it is likely that she will either require plating or TENS nailing to her forearm fractures and plating or TENS nailing of the femoral fracture.

Had the story changed or the possibility of non-accidental injury been raised what other factors from the history and injury pattern might confirm this?

Fractures with soft-tissue injuries constitute the majority of manifestations of physical abuse in children. Fracture and injury patterns vary with age and development, and NAI is intrinsically related to the mobility of the child. No fracture in isolation is pathognomonic of NAI, but specific abuse-related injuries include multiple fractures, particularly at various stages of healing, metaphyseal corner and bucket-handle fractures and fractures of ribs. Isolated or multiple rib fractures, irrespective of location, have the highest specificity for NAI. Other fractures with a high specificity for abuse include those of the scapula, lateral end of the clavicle, vertebrae and complex skull fractures.

Her parents want to know how long fractures take to heal. What will you tell them?

Fractures in adults typically take 3-months to 'heal' (i.e. cortices are congruent)

and bone remodelling continues beyond 6-months. Radiographic evidence of callus formation is visible on radiographs at around 4-weeks and patients are usually mobilised between weeks 4 to 6. In children healing is slightly quicker and the parents can expect bone healing to take 3-6 weeks.

SUMMARY

The ABCDEs of assessment are the same in children and adults, the anatomical and physiological variances require consideration for simple fluid resuscitation and drug administration or more complex interventions (ie. soft tissues in an infant´s oropharynx are larger than in an adult and make visualization of the larynx difficult for intubation). Polytraumas with distracting injuries can be particularly challenging especially with children or reduced GCS when communication is tricky. Follow ATLS protocols, identify life-threatening injuries and perform a full secondary survey to avoid missing any other injuries.

TOP TIPS

➕ Remember to be conscious of non-accidental injury in children.

➕ Early involvement of senior surgeon or if available paediatric surgeon.

➕ Consider that the child's skeleton is incompletely calcified and therefore more pliable than an adult. For this reason the fracture of a bone requires a high energy trauma.

➕ Broselow paediatric emergency tape can be useful and is a length-based resuscitation tape for fluid volumes, drug doses and equipment size that is often kept in emergency departments.

CLINICAL

4 MANAGEMENT

MANAGEMENT

4.1 Dealing with a Complaint

Scenario

You are assisting in a total knee replacement and are lumbered with the task of supporting the leg. You mention that this would be much easier if the patient wasn't so fat. You realise in a moment of horror that the patient is under spinal anaesthesia and heard your comment.

How would you approach this scenario?

Seek information: It may be obvious that the patient is upset. Apologise for your remark and ask whether she is happy for you to continue to assist. Tell her you will speak to her after the operation, as this must take priority.

Patient safety: There is no direct threat to patient safety, but you have compromised the patient's trust in yourself and the profession. If your behaviour has made the patient feel unsafe, you should find somebody else to assist.

Initiative: Visit the patient at the earliest opportunity after the operation. Explore her concerns surrounding the incident. Hopefully these can be settled with an apology and reassurance that it will not happen again.

Escalate: Discuss the incident with the operating surgeon. You should also inform your clinical supervisor who will be able to offer you advice and support in case the patient registers a complaint.

Support: If you are unable to settle the problem yourself you should ask somebody the patient trusts to speak with her. Ideally this person should be the operating surgeon. If the patient remains unhappy and wishes to make a formal complaint, you should help put her in touch with the appropriate person.

What are the key issues?

This is an embarrassing situation to be in. It is important to focus on making the patient safe (i.e. finishing the operation) before dedicating your efforts to resolving the complaint itself.

Despite attempts by yourself and the surgeon to allay the situation, the patient remains upset and wishes to make a complaint against you. What do you do now?

Most complaints can be resolved informally. Nevertheless, the patient is within her rights to make a formal complaint if she wishes. You should give her the contact details for the patient advice and liaison service (PALS). Make sure she knows that this will not affect the care she is given. Again, the surgeon and your supervisor should be informed.

What future impact may the event have on the patient?

The patient may lose trust in you, the consultant or the profession. If she develops a complication post-operatively, she may avoid attending and suffer serious consequences.

MANAGEMENT

The patient's husband has appeared on the ward. He is angry about your comment. What do you do?

Gain the patient's consent before you discuss anything with the husband. Use a similar approach, trying to talk the husband down and involving colleagues as necessary. If he remains unhappy, he is able to lodge a complaint.

What would differ if the complainant had learning difficulties?

The complaint must be taken just as seriously. Encourage the patient to involve their family/carers. Again, try to resolve the issue informally. There are no restrictions about who can make a formal complaint. Therefore, you should make it possible for the patient, their family or carers to complain if they so wish.

What is the patient advice and liaison service?

It serves as a point of contact for patients and their families, offering confidential advice, support and information. All formal complaints should be lodged via PALS. You have fifteen days to respond to a formal complaint made against you.

What happens next?

Usually the complaints procedure stops after your letter of apology/explanation of events. If the patient is not satisfied, the complaint can be escalated via PALS to the clinical director. Occasionally the local ombudsman will need to be involved.

When would the General Medical Council get involved?

The GMC deals with the most serious complaints which cannot be resolved at a lower level. This means complaints that might require a doctor's registration to be restricted or removed to protect the public and uphold public confidence in the medical profession.

SUMMARY

Many surgeons will receive a complaint at some point in their career. In fact, 1 in 64 doctors is investigated by the General Medical Council following a complaint. Getting a complaint can be demoralising, but an open and honest approach invariably leads to better patient satisfaction whilst protecting your integrity.

TOP TIPS

➕ Try to resolve the complaint informally first.

➕ Do not deny a patient the right to complain, even if it is about you.

➕ Consider the impact on both the complainant and the defendant.

MANAGEMENT

4.2 Drunk Colleague

> **Scenario**
>
> You are assisting the registrar who is about to perform an incision and drainage in theatre. You notice her hands are shaking and she smells strongly of alcohol.

How would you approach this scenario?

Seek information: You already have reason to suspect the registrar is drunk, and must act on this quickly. Seeking further information would waste time.

Patient safety: The registrar must be removed from theatre and kept away from other clinical areas. This should be achieved in the least confrontational manner. Initially you should politely ask her yourself. Failing this, involve a senior member of your team or, if necessary, another team to try and convince her to leave.

Initiative: Ensure the safety of the registrar by booking her a taxi home. Endeavour to find somebody from your team or a neighbouring team to cover the list. Check whether the registrar has had contact with any other patients today; if so make sure they are safe.

Escalate: The situation needs to be escalated to the consultant in charge of the operating list, so alternative arrangements can be made. It is also important to tell the registrar's clinical supervisor. Avoid telling anyone who does not need to be involved.

Support: This may be a one-off episode or part of an enduring alcohol problem; either way the registrar will need support. The list may be cancelled if nobody is able to cover. If so, the patient(s) should be offered an apology. Do explain that the registrar is unwell but avoid mentioning anything incriminating for the registrar. Support the team who may need to take on extra duties in the registrar's absence.

What are the key issues?

This scenario requires you to think about the safety of both the patient and the registrar. The registrar have personal problems which led to the event and, unless offered appropriate support, could result in further episodes.

The registrar's mother died last week. How does this change matters?

The alcoholism is likely to be a recent problem related to the bereavement, but it is difficult to predict how long it will last. The registrar will need counselling for both the alcohol problem and the bereavement. The situation may be resolved by giving the registrar compassionate leave until she is safe to return.

What would you tell the patient?

Do not tell the patient that the registrar is drunk, as this will only serve to worry the patient and damage their trust in the profession. Instead, say the registrar is unwell and the operation must be cancelled/delayed for the patient's safety.

MANAGEMENT

Who else could you tell?

You have been placed in an awkward position and are likely to need support and advice yourself. Speak to a senior colleague whom you trust, such as your clinical supervisor. If you belong to a medical indemnity organisation, call them for advice.

The registrar offers to pay you £100 to keep quiet. What do you do?

Decline the bribe. Be open with the registrar; tell them why you must escalate the matter for everybody's safety (including your own). Explain that you have the registrar's best interests at heart. Promise not to tell anyone who does not need to know, such as the other trainees.

What would you do if you heard your colleagues talking about your drunk registrar in the doctors' mess?

Do not join in. Try to dispel the gossip and remind your colleagues of their professional responsibility. There is nothing to be gained from personally blaming the person who spread the news. You should mention the registrar's bereavement to those she trusts, so they can offer their support.

How do you expect your senior to manage the registrar once you have escalated?

The consultant must make a decision about the gravity of the situation. The situation will be escalated to the appropriate level (clinical director to medical director to chief executive to GMC). The registrar may be given a warning, or referred to the GMC for suspension.

How would the situation differ if the proposed operation was a hemicolectomy rather than an incision and drainage?

The registrar is unsafe to perform any surgery, however simple the procedure. You are more likely to find someone to cover the abscess drainage than the more specialist hemicolectomy. In fact, you may even be competent to do it yourself.

If the registrar had been taking illegal drugs, should you tell the police?

Think about what this would achieve. It would be better to get the registrar help for her drug problem rather than punishment. Your duty is to escalate as before. If it is decided that the police must be involved for any reason, you would not be expected to do this yourself.

MANAGEMENT

SUMMARY

Alcohol abuse is a common problem within the medical profession. As always, safety is paramount. This includes considering the safety of the patient, the registrar, the team and yourself. Protect yourself by escalating to your seniors, even if the registrar asks you not to.

TOP TIPS

 Approach the situation sensitively.

 Show humanity; your role is to support the registrar not to accuse.

4.3 | Self-Discharge

Scenario

A patient with suspected appendicitis has been waiting 6 hours to be seen as you have been busy assisting in theatre. She is angry about being kept waiting and is threatening to self-discharge.

How would you approach this scenario?

Seek information: See this patient as a priority. Explore her ideas, concerns and expectations regarding admission. Identify any underlying reasons for her to self-discharge.

Patient Safety: A diagnosis of appendicitis needs to be managed promptly. Similarly, she may have a ruptured ectopic pregnancy. Either of these diagnoses could have serious consequences if the patient self discharges without treatment.

Initiative: Explain why self-discharge would be inadvisable and try to persuade her to stay. Offer reassurance that ultimately this is her decision, which will be respected.

Escalate: Inform the registrar and consultant on call, who may be able to convince the patient to stay. If the patient still refuses to stay despite attempts to persuade her, you must let her go.

Support: Reassure the patient that the hospital is always open and that you will gladly see her again if she changes her mind.

MANAGEMENT

Why is the patient reluctant to stay in hospital?

It may be that she is bored of waiting, in which case you may be able to change her mind by seeing her promptly. Is she afraid of hospital for some reason?

The patient has attended with her boyfriend, who is telling her to hurry up and sign the self-discharge form. Does this change your management?

Yes, you must see the patient alone to ensure she is not being coerced into self-discharge. Reiterate that it is her decision, not the boyfriend's.

What if this is her third attendance in as many days?

This should alert you to a social problem; possibly domestic abuse. Take care to reassure her the hospital is a safe place. Escalate to your safeguarding lead.

Can she still self-discharge?

If the patient is able to understand and retain the information given, weigh up the risks, and communicate her decision, then she has capacity. Ensure she is free from coercion, which may affect her ability to weigh up the risks. You must respect any decision made by a patient with capacity, however unwise it may seem.

What if she absconds before signing the self-discharge form?

Patients often do! In this case, make sure you document any discussions had with the patient. The self-discharge form confirms that the patient has capacity and understands the potential implications of refusing medical advice. Finally, it states follow up arrangements. It is not a legal document, but protects you by placing the responsibility on the patient.

What if the patient leaves before you have even seen them?

You should take reasonable steps to ensure the patient is safe. This may involve contacting the patient by telephone to discuss the aforementioned issues. If you are concerned about a vulnerable patient, escalate to the local safeguarding lead and inform the patient's GP.

Is there a limit to how many times a patient can self-discharge?

No. Patients who recurrently self-discharge should be offered the same treatment as anyone else. Although you may feel like the patient is wasting your time, be careful you do not make them feel unwelcome. Be acutely aware of any concomitant social problems leading to this behaviour.

For what reasons do patients self-discharge?

More than ten percent of patients attending accident and emergency self-discharge before being seen. Of all A&E self-discharges, about half are related to drugs or alcohol. Other social issues play a part and these patients should therefore be considered vulnerable.

MANAGEMENT

SUMMARY

This scenario pivots on the issue of capacity. Take the necessary steps to enable the patient to reach their own decision. Be honest about the consequences of refusing medical advice, which may in this case include death. Welcome the patient to return at any stage in the future.

TOP TIPS

 Respect the decision of the patient.

 Use 'safety nets' and make sure there are no barriers to the patient's return if she changes her mind.

4.4 | Struggling Colleague

Scenario

One of your fellow core surgical trainees appears to be struggling at work. He looks stressed and, despite staying late most days, often leaves his jobs unfinished.

How would you approach this scenario?

Seek information: Find out why your colleague is struggling. Has the workload been delegated unfairly towards him? Is he new to the job? Does he have some personal issues which are distracting him from his work?

Patient safety: There may be a threat to patient safety if your colleague is tired from working late each day. Also, if he is stressed he may lack concentration and again jeopardise patient safety.

Initiative: Speak to your colleague to find out where the issues lie. Offer to help out with the jobs, and let him shadow you to see how you manage the workload more effectively. If there are temporary problems outside of work, be flexible and try to cover some of the clinical duties between yourself and the rest of the team.

Escalate: If you are concerned about the safety of your patients or your colleague you should escalate to the consultant.

Support: Support your colleague with his workload and any concurrent personal problems. Advise him to speak to his on supervisor or a counsellor if appropriate. If your team is taking on extra work as a result of your struggling colleague, support them through this too.

MANAGEMENT

What are the key issues?

There may be many reasons why your colleague is struggling with his work: is there too much of it? Is he unsupported by the team? Does he need some more training? Are there problems outside of work? For the safety of the patients and there wellbeing of your colleague, these issues need to be sorted sooner rather than later, before he burns out.

You discover your colleague is going through a divorce. How do you handle the situation now?

Your colleague is going through a difficult time in his personal life and this is impacting on his work. This sort of problem will not resolve overnight and he may benefit from some time off work. If this is not possible, reduced hours or duties may help. It is not your job to counsel him through the divorce, but you could point him in the direction of someone who can help.

Your colleague denies anything is wrong and refuses to change his working hours. What can you do?

Work may be a good distraction for your colleague so, unless he is unsafe to work, he should be allowed to continue if he wishes. Make sure your team is aware of the situation so they can continue to support him. Let your colleague know he can change his mind if he needs to take time off.

What support is available for a struggling colleague such as this?

Within the workplace, your colleague can speak to a trusted team member such as his supervisor. He could attend occupational health department or his own GP. There are many counselling services available, both privately and on the NHS, which could help him manage the divorce. Independent charities such as Relate offer relationship help and can be accessed online, over the telephone or in person.

You suspect your colleague is abusing alcohol as a coping mechanism. What do you do now?

Once again, patient safety is paramount and you must take the above steps to ensure this. You will have to inform the consultant about your colleague's drinking so appropriate measures can be taken to protect the patients and the colleague himself. Although it may seem like you are adding to his troubles, you would be doing no one a favour by keeping quiet about this. Approach the situation sensitively and be non-judgmental.

How do you recognise a struggling colleague?

Stress manifests itself in different ways in different people. Some people become irritable and argumentative, whilst others may withdraw to avoid confrontation. Signs may be very subtle or as obvious as a mid-ward breakdown. Everyone in this career will face stress at some point; be vigilant so you can offer support at an early stage.

MANAGEMENT

How do you manage stress?

Thinking about how you handle stress may help you empathise with your colleague and even suggest coping strategies to him. Firstly, you need to identify when you are stressed then, depending on the situation, you will have various coping mechanisms. These may include sharing your problems with colleagues, friends and family; socialising, exercise and focussing on your hobbies.

How do you handle stress at work?

Techniques include anticipating and preparing for stressful situations - such as a crash call; being organised and efficient; utilising other team members; taking regular breaks; handing over unfinished tasks where appropriate; asking for help when needed; and having a positive team spirit.

How can you help support your team through a stressful time?

A good relationship with your team members is fundamental. Encourage a culture of openness. Be approachable and accessible. When a colleague requires you to take on extra duties for them, do so graciously. Organising events for the team outside of work can help build a successful team.

SUMMARY

You are likely to encounter a struggling colleague or indeed, be that person, during the course of your career. The key issues to consider will be the safety and wellbeing of the patients, the colleague and the team. Involve yourself and other relevant parties as necessary, but beware the fine balance between helping and interfering.

TOP TIPS

 Support your colleague as you would wish to be supported - one day it may be you that is struggling.

MANAGEMENT

4.5 Refusal of Treatment

Scenario

You are the general surgical SHO on call. A patient with a background of schizophrenia has been admitted with severe right iliac fossa pain and has been diagnosed with appendicitis. They are planned for an appendicectomy on the emergency list. You have been asked to obtain consent from the patient however the patient is adamant he does not want an operation.

How would you approach this situation?

Seek Information: You need to be confident in receiving consent for this procedure, in so much that you understand the procedure and the associated risks and benefits. You need to ascertain what the patient understands by the procedure being proposed and their reasons for refusing consent.

Patient Safety: By refusing to consent to theatre this patient is endangering their health and being put a risk of complications such as sepsis and potentially death.

Initiative: You can identify the patient's main concerns and reasons for refusing consent. If you are appropriately familiar with the procedure and its associated risks then you may be able to answer any questions and put at ease any cause for anxiety. You could also assess the patient's capacity to consent for theatre. However, it should not be assumed that just because a patient is making the assumed wrong decision that they do not have capacity.

Escalate: Due to the severity of potential consequences of refusing surgery it would then be appropriate to escalate this situation to your seniors if the patient continues to have reservations. By involving more members of the team, including the lead surgeon, this may help the patient feel more comfortable about the surgery.

Support: It may also be helpful to ask the patient if they wish to discuss their options with relatives or friends and offer to have further discussions with them once they have had further opportunity to digest the information and may have formulated further questions. If the patient continues to refuse to consent and they are deemed to have capacity then it is important to continue to treat and manage their symptoms to the best of your team's ability without operative intervention.

What are the key issues in this scenario?

The key issues here are of consent, and the capacity to give consent.

The patient's sister then arrives on the ward and wants the patient to go ahead with the surgery but they continue to refuse to give consent. His sister then questions whether his decision making can be depended upon due to the patient's mental health issues.

What information about the patient's condition can be disclosed to their sister?

You should establish with the patient what information they want you to share, who with, and in what circumstances.

The patient's medical condition can only be discussed with his sister with the patient's consent. If the patient does not wish for the details to be given to his sister then the principles of patient confidentially should be explained to the relative and these should be maintained despite her relation to the patient.

Does a diagnosis of a mental illness imply that there is a lack of capacity?

No. Mental illness and capacity are two separate entities. However, in some cases a psychiatric condition may affect someone's capacity but this should not be assumed. If there is any doubt a capacity assessment should be conducted.

What is meant by capacity?

You must work on the presumption that every adult patient has the capacity to make decisions about their care and to decide whether to agree to, or refuse, an examination, investigation or treatment. You must only regard a patient as lacking capacity once it is clear that, having been given all appropriate help and support, they cannot understand, retain, use or weigh up the information needed to make that decision, or communicate their wishes.

The person giving consent needs to have capacity to give the consent. To have capacity one must be able to retain the information, understand the information, weight up the information to make an informed decision and the be able to communicate their decision.

How is capacity assessed?

You must assess a patient's capacity to make a particular decision at the time it needs to be made. You must not assume that because a patient lacks capacity to make a decision on a particular occasion, they lack capacity to make any decisions at all, or will not be able to make decisions in the future.

You must take account of the advice on assessing capacity in the Codes of Practice that accompany the Mental Capacity Act 2005 and the Adults with Incapacity (Scotland) Act 2000 and other relevant guidance. If your assessment is that the patient's capacity is borderline, you must be able to show that it is more likely than not that they lack capacity.

If your assessment leaves you in doubt about the patient's capacity to make a decision, you should seek advice from:

- Nursing staff or others involved in the patient's care, or those close to the patient, who may be aware of the patient's usual ability to make decisions and their particular communication needs.

- Colleagues with relevant specialist experience, such as psychiatrists, neurologists, or speech and language therapists.

If you are still unsure about the patient's capacity to make a decision, you must seek legal advice with a view to asking a court to determine capacity.

What is involved in the consent procedure?

With regards to consent there are two people involved: the person giving consent (the patient) and the person receiving consent (the surgeon). The person receiving consent should understand the procedure as well as reasons for it being conducted and any associated common and rare but serious complications.

For how long does consent last?

Each time consent is sought it is for a particular situation with a particular patient in particular circumstances. Each time anyone of these changes the issue of consent should be revisited. For example, if the patient's condition changes this may make the need for surgery more urgent and complications of refusing surgery more severe or it may mean the the patient is now more unstable making the risks of an anaesthetic and surgery higher. A patient can also withdraw consent at any time, whether there is a change in the situation or not, and this should be explained when explaining the consent procedure.

What can be done if the patient continues to refuse to consent?

As a medical professional you can encourage on going conversations with the patient and try and answer any questions that they have or, if appropriate, assure any anxieties that they have about the procedure. You should also ensure that they have a full grasp on the potential consequences of not consenting for theatre. However, it is important that you remain professional and do not try and intimidate or coerce the patient into consenting. At the end of the day it needs to be the patient's decision.

You must respect a competent patient's decision to refuse an investigation or treatment, even if you think their decision is wrong or irrational. You may advise the patient of your clinical opinion, but you must not put pressure on them to accept your advice. You must be careful that your words and actions do not imply judgement of the patient or their beliefs and values.

Can anyone else consent for a patient?

The only situations were someone other than the patient can consent on their behalf is if the patient is a minor (under 16 years old and deemed not to have competence) or the patient lacks capacity. A lack of capacity may be due to a chronic condition (either medical or psychiatric) or a temporary, reversible condition, for example, a patient being unconscious because of a head trauma or due to profound sepsis. A next of kin can consent for a patient, or if they are not available a consent form 4 can be completed by two medical professionals, one being of consultant grade. A procedure can also be carried out without consent in an emergency setting where the patients is too acutely unwell to give consent and it is believed that delaying treatment could be life-threatening.

SUMMARY

The issues surrounding consent are complicated and can become emotive especially when it is regarding a patient refusing life saving treatment. It can be difficult to say in an interview that you would continue not to treat someone when they will potentially die from lack of intervention but you must stick your guns. Treating someone without consent is assault. The issue of capacity is also very important and should be assessed by someone trained in doing so. It should never be assumed that because you believe someone is making the wrong decision that they must not have capacity.

TOP TIPS

✚ Have a clear idea in your head of who can gain consent and what you need to know in order to do so.

✚ Also be confident in the attributes needed to have capacity.

✚ If you get handed a complicated scenario just stick to these principles - even if it means a poor outcome for the patient.

MANAGEMENT

4.6 | Explaining DNAR

Scenario

You are the orthopaedic SHO covering the neck of femur unit. One of the patients has developed new left sided weakness and dysphasia. Following medical review and investigations they have been diagnosed with a CVA. The patient also has a past medical history of AF, COPD and CKD. They are physiologically frail. It is the opinion of the medical and surgical teams that attempts at CPR would be inappropriate and likely futile in this patient. You have been asked to discuss completing a DNACPR form with the patient and their daughter.

How would you approach this situation?

Seek Information: Prior to having a conversation with the patient and their family it would be sensible to review the medical notes and investigations so that you are completely familiar with the patient and their medical state. It is then useful to begin the discussion by asking how much the patient and their daughter knows about what has happened during this inpatient stay. You should then make sure that they are happy to discuss what has been happening in further detail - some patients do not what to know the ins and outs of how unwell they are.

Patient Safety: In this scenario it would be prudent to check with the patient that they are happy to have this discussion with their daughter present. Most patients will be grateful for some family support, however others may not want relatives knowing details of their medical state.

Initiative: These types of conversations should ideally be had somewhere quiet and so if possible a quiet room should be used. If the patient is too unwell to move from their bed then it may be an idea to ask a relative to come in outside of visiting times so that the ward is not noisy and full of other visitors when having this type of discussion.

Escalate: This could be viewed by some as a 'life or death' type of discussion and some may feel uncomfortable if they view this type of decision as having come from a 'junior doctor.' It should be explained that DNACRP decisions come following a team discussion, including the patient's consultant. However, if the patient or relative are still uneasy then you could arrange a discussion with a more senior member of the team. It should also be explained that this may take more time as senior surgeons are often not available to come to the ward at short notice due to theatre and clinic commitments.

Support: Patients and relatives often do not take in all that has been explained especially if they have been given a large amount of information, particularly medical details which will be foreign to them. It would be useful to reassure them that should any further questions arise or they want to rediscuss something at a later date then a member of the team will always be able to come and have a further discussion.

What are the key issues in this scenario?

The main issues in this scenario are deciding which patients would not be appropriate for attempts at CPR, who can make those decisions and whether putting a DNACPR form in place can be refused.

When broaching the subject of DNACPR the patient's daughter becomes very anxious and asks whether you are going to stop treating her mum and put her on the 'death pathway.' Because of these concerns she is not happy with a DNACPR form being put in place. How would you broach these concerns of the daughter about a DNACPR form?

Firstly, it is important that you fully and clearly explain what a DNACPR form entails. You should be explicit in saying that it does imply a withdrawal of treatment and that you and the medical team will continue to treat her mum with anything that is believed to be effective and of benefit to her. It should be explained that a DNACPR form only comes into effect when the patient's heart stops. In this case, it is the opinion of the medical team that were this to happen it would not be something that could be reversed; that given her age, multiple medical conditions and recent trauma, that trying to get her heart to restart would either be futile or the effects of her other organs, including her brain, having had no circulation for any period of time would be significant and mean that her mother would not regain any form of quality of life.

What would you explain about the 'death pathway'?

In recent years there has been much press attention about the management of dying patients, with particular reference to the 'Liverpool Care Pathway.' Many medical professionals believe that the issues around the LCP were not handled well and were portrayed unfairly in the media. However it is important not to get bogged down in the politics of healthcare. You should firstly ask the daughter what she understands by the term 'death pathway' and then explain the facts. Care of the dying pathways are for patients who it is felt are dying and that any treatment at all would be ineffective or just prolong the inevitable. In that situation the focus of the medical team is on symptom management rather than the active treatment of any medical conditions.

What is the difference between DNACPR and care of the dying pathways?

Most pertinently, a DNACPR form does not involve the withdrawal of treatment, they are put in place for patients in whom it is felt that any attempts at restarting their heart would be futile or would not restore any form of quality of life. The emphasis of the medical team then switches from treating medical conditions to symptom control, for example pain relief and relaxants.

Who can put a DNACPR form in place?

A DNACPR form can be signed by any doctor who is fully registered with the GMC (ie anyone higher than FY1). They should then be further signed by a

MANAGEMENT

senior doctor (registrar or higher) at a later date to confirm that the whole team is in agreement.

The overall clinical responsibility for decisions about CPR, including DNACPR decisions, rests with the most senior clinician responsible for the person's care as defined explicitly by local policy.

For which patients can you put a DNACPR form in place?

Technically any patient. However, it is good medical practice for this to be a team decision. If it is for a patient who you review on an oncall shift then you should inform other medical professions, for example the medical registrar, and also discuss it with the patient's usual nursing team to gage what they feel is appropriate. The patient's named medical team should then be informed at the earliest opportunity.

If cardiac or respiratory arrest is an expected part of the dying process and CPR will not be successful, making and recording an advance decision not to attempt CPR will help to ensure that the patient dies in a dignified and peaceful manner. It may also help to ensure that the patient's last hours or days are spent in their preferred place of care by, for example, avoiding emergency admission from a community setting to hospital. These management plans are called do not attempt CPR (DNACPR) orders, or do not attempt resuscitation or allow natural death decisions.

Is a DNACPR form permanent?

No. A DNACPR form can be taken out of the notes at any stage. This can be discussed with family, for example, when an elderly patient is severely unwell from an infection and it is felt that with the current insult, if they were to arrest, they would not have the physical reserve to be resuscitated. However, if the treatment for their infection is successful and they recover, they may then become physiologically strong enough for an attempt at CPR to be appropriate. If a patient with a DNACPR form is nearing discharge a team decision should also be made as to whether the form continues in the community ie a 'community DNACPR form.'

Can a patient or relative refuse a DNACPR form?

Technically no, and this can lead to some difficult conversations. At a basic level performing attempts at CPR is a medical intervention and the decision to perform an intervention or treatment lies solely with the medical team. For example, it is the decision of the surgeon whether they feel an operative intervention is appropriate or not, if they feel it is not then a patient does not have the right to demand an operation. However, as CPR is dealing with people at the cusp of death these types of decisions can become far more emotive, particularly for the patients and relatives involved. There has also been recent media coverage about these issues. This has lead to emphasis being put on discussions about DNACPR happening prior to a form being put in place which is important. The main way of avoiding confrontation is through good communication and early involvement of the patient and relatives so that they have been with you through the entire decision making process.

SUMMARY

The key to DNACPR discussions is good communication. As well as yourself and the patient, there are often relatives present (usually due to the frailty of the patients involved in these discussions) and it can also be useful to have their named nurse with you as well, as they spend the most time with the patients and relatives. It is important to be clear on what will happen when a DNACPR form is put in place and this can also be a good opportunity to discuss in broader terms what level of care you feel would be appropriate for this patient to be escalated to if they deteriorate on their current treatment, for example would they be a candidate for NIV or HDU, or are they purely for ward-based level of care.

TOP TIPS

➕ Start any discussion with what the patient and relatives understand by what has happened so far during their admission. Then give a brief summary of what you understand has happened and this can then segway into what the plans are for the future and how far treatment should be escalated.

➕ Be explicit that a DNACPR form does not mean withdrawal of treatment.

➕ Have team discussions so that you can reassure the patient and relatives that all parties involved in their care feel that this is appropriate.

➕ Offer to have further discussions if they need more clarification or think of further questions.

MANAGEMENT

4.7 | Patient Confidentiality

Scenario

You have been conducting an audit of patients recently admitted to your surgical ward. You saved the patient data on a memory stick. Later that week the memory stick falls out of your bag whilst paying for a coffee in the outpatient department. The stick is found by a patient who then looks at the contents in order to identify the owner. They then hand the USB stick into the Patient Advice and Liaison Service and explain that they have seen the confidential patient data saved on the device.

How would you approach this situation?

Seek Information: You should make youe supervisors (educational and clinical) aware of this situation. Not only is this important for your duty of candour but they can also offer you support and advice. An error has been made by you but they may be able to offer advice as to how best to rectify the situation.

Patient Safety: Patient confidentially has been broken and the extent of this needs to be clearly established. It should be found out how much of the information was seen by the patient and what details were seen. The individuals who are then affected should be informed and apologised to.

Initiative: You should also take this opportunity to reflect on the situation, including what you have learnt and what you would do differently. You could also undertake further education on patient confidentiality, for example e-learning.

Escalate: It is possible that this breach in patient confidentiality will be escalated through the ranks of seniority from PALS who were initially alerted to the breach. It would therefore be prudent of you to escalate this situation through your seniors and involve your supervisors at the earliest opportunity.

Support: Relating to the previous point, it is important to inform your supervisors and there may also be further support you can access from human resources and those involved with you training programme.

What are the key issues in this scenario?

The main issue here is obviously that of patient confidentiality which has been breached. This scenario also highlights the issue of doctor's candour and being honest and open about mistakes that have been made and then showing what you have learnt from the incident and measures that have been put in place to avoid that mistake from being repeated.

The patients who had their confidentiality breached by having their details viewed on the USB stick are informed and one patient is wishing to make a formal complaint and wants the situation escalated to higher management.

MANAGEMENT

What is the complaints process within the NHS?

The NHS has a complaints procedure that is designed to be as patient focused as possible and investigate complaints effectively and efficiently. It is a two stage process; the first is called local resolution. With local resolution you can complain to either the provider or the commissioner of the health service you are unhappy about.

- The provider is the organisation that provides the service to the patient, for instance a GP, dentist, pharmacist or a hospital.
- NHS England is the commissioner or purchaser of primary care i.e GPs, dentists, opticians, pharmacy and some specialised services.
- Clinical commissioning groups commission hospital services, mental health services, out of hours services and 111 services amongst others.

The complaint will then be investigated and the result communicated back to the complainant.

If you are not content with their reply, the next step is to ask the parliamentary and health service ombudsman (PHSO) to review the complaint and how it has been handled.

If questions are then raised about your professionalism how is this dealt with?

NHS trusts will manage complaints at a hospital level by the channels laid out by NHS England as above. However, if there is a question over an individuals practice then a complaint can be made to their regulatory body. In the case of doctors this is the general medical council.

The purpose of the professional regulators is to protect and promote the safety of the public. They do this by setting standards of behaviour, education and ethics that health professionals must meet. They deal with concerns about professionals who are unfit to practise due to poor health, misconduct or poor performance. Regulators register health professionals who are fit to practise in the UK, and can remove a professional from the register and stop them from practising if it's in the interests of public safety.

What aspect of GMC guidance has been breached here?

Good medical practice (2013) makes clear that patients have a right to expect that information about them will be held in confidence by their doctors. The GMC has published Confidentiality (2009) which sets out the principles of confidentiality and respect for patients' privacy that doctors are expected to understand and follow.

What resources can you utilise to offer support and further information in this scenario?

If you are subject to investigation or action by the GMC or other body you should contact your medical defence organisation straight away. They can offer you advice and legal support if appropriate. If you are not a member of a defence organisation, you could contact the British Medical Association who can provide expert advice and support.

MANAGEMENT

Alternatively, you can get your own legal advice, at your own expense. Legal aid is not available to doctors being investigated under GMC procedures and you cannot claim costs from the other parties involved. The NHS also has a duty of care towards its staff and your employer should offer you access to occupational health services and should ensure that proper confidentiality procedures are put in place so as to limit any damage from malicious complaints.

What do you understand by the duty of candour?

Secondary care providers registered with CQC in England are now subject to a statutory duty of candour, introduced in November 2014.

Doctors have had a professional duty of candour for many years. In its core guidance for doctors, Good medical practice (2013) paragraph 55, the GMC says:
"You must be open and honest with patients if things go wrong. If a patient under your care has suffered harm or distress, you should:

- Put matters right *(if that is possible)*
- Offer an apology
- Explain fully and promptly what has happened and the likely short-term and long-term effects."

The new statutory duty of candour was introduced for NHS bodies in England (trusts, foundation trusts and special health authorities) from 27 November 2014.
The obligations associated with the statutory duty of candour are contained in regulation 20 of The Health and Social Care Act 2008 (Regulated Activities).

How should the patient confidential information have been stored?

Patient confidential information can be stored either on an NHS server system or on an encrypted USB stick - this can be obtained from your NHS hospital.

Should the patients have consented to you taking this information?

No. You are not required to gain patient consent for information being used in audit as long as there are no patient identifiable factors available in the reports. As laid out in GMC guidance:

When disclosing information about a patient, you must:
- Use anonymised or coded information if practicable and if it will serve the purpose
- Be satisfied that the patient:
  - Has ready access to information that explains that their personal information might be disclosed for the sake of their own care, or for local clinical audit, and that they can object, and
  - Has not objected

When are doctors allowed to break confidentiality?

Confidentiality is an important duty, but it is not absolute. You can disclose personal information if:

- It is required by law e.g to a police officer or the courts
- The patient consents – either implicitly for the sake of their own care or expressly for other purposes e.g. on patient information leaflets or websites
- It is justified in the public interest

SUMMARY

This is a serious topic with potentially disastrous consequences for any doctors involved. The legislation and GMC guidance surrounding confidentiality and complaints procedures can be complicated and lengthy but having a knowledge of the key principles should be sufficient. An important aspect is to emphasise the necessity about being open and honest about any mistakes.

TOP TIPS

➕ Read the summaries of guidance on confidentiality outlined by the GMC so that you are familiar with the key principles.

➕ Mention that you would discuss with the affected patients at the earliest opportunity.

➕ Have a plan for how you would move forward from this, for example, reflection, further learning and possibly planning teaching sessions for you and your peers. This would demonstrate duty of candour and allowing others to learn from your mistakes will benefit the medical profession and patients in the future.

MANAGEMENT

4.8 | Consent

> ### Scenario
>
> You are the general surgery SHO on call and are called down to A&E to review a child with suspected appendicitis. After reviewing the patient and their investigations you agree with the diagnosis and explain to the parents the recommendation for surgical management. However, the parents immediately refuse to give consent for the surgery and express a strong belief that alternative medicines will treat their child more effectively and with less risk.

How would you approach this situation?

Seek information: Firstly, review the patient and their investigations to make sure that you are confident in the diagnosis. Explore in depth the parent's reasons for refusing surgery and explain to the best of your abilities the surgical team's reasons for wanting to proceed with an operation.

Patient Safety: The health of the child is potentially at risk in this situation. You should make sure that the parents are fully aware of the severity of the potential complications of not proceeding to theatre, including overwhelming sepsis and possible death. If the parents still refuse consent this may need to be escalated to go against their refusal of consent and this will be discussed in detail later.

Initiative: It may help to have some statistics readily available with regards to risks of surgery vs risks of non-operative intervention with appendicitis. This may help strengthen the surgical team's point of view during discussion with the parents. You could also do some research into the evidence of alternative medicine treatments for appendicitis and the success rates (or lack thereof).

Escalate: This situation has the potential to become complicated and it is important you involve your seniors early on. Having senior input may also make the parents more confident in the surgical team's proposed treatment.

Support: Again, having full team input is necessary in these cases and it is important to make sure that the whole team is giving consistent information to the parents. If this needs to be escalated, with the surgical team aiming to go against the parents' wishes then legal teams should be involved in a timely fashion.

What are the key issues in this scenario?

This scenario is based around the issue of consent. As this involves a minor who is not consenting for themselves this is also a situation where the wishes of a parent or guardian can be gone against if it is deemed in the patient's best interests.

The parents continue to refuse to consent to an operation despite further discussions with the Consultant surgeon. The patient's pain then worsens, they start to show signs of sepsis and there is a suspicion that they may now have a ruptured appendix. The need

for surgery becomes more pressing and the surgical and A&E teams believe it may become necessary to go against the parents' wishes and proceed with operative intervention.

If a patient is refusing to consent for themselves then healthcare professionals can not go against that. How is this situation different?

In this situation it is not the patient making the decision. It is their parent's decision that is impacting upon the patient, with potential adverse effects. As such, it is possible for the parents' wishes to be gone against and for medical professionals to provide consent if they believe not doing so will have severe adverse implications for the patient's health.

How would you assess whether the patient can consent for themselves rather than requiring parental consent?

The capacity to consent depends more on young people's ability to understand and weigh up options than on age. When assessing a young person's capacity to consent, you should bear in mind that:

- At 16 a young person can be presumed to have the capacity to consent
- A young person under 16 may have the capacity to consent, depending on their maturity and ability to understand what is involved.

It is important that you assess maturity and understanding on an individual basis and with regard to the complexity and importance of the decision to be made. You should remember that a young person who has the capacity to consent to a straightforward, relatively risk-free treatment may not necessarily have the capacity to consent to complex treatment involving high risks or serious consequences. The capacity to consent can also be affected by their physical and emotional development and by changes in their health and treatment.

What do you understand by Gillick Competence and Fraser Guidelines?

Gillick competency and Fraser guidelines refer to a legal case which looked specifically at whether doctors should be able to give contraceptive advice or treatment to children under 16 without parental consent. But since then, they have been more widely used to help assess whether a child has the maturity to make their own decisions and to understand the implications of those decisions.

In 1982 Mrs Victoria Gillick took her local health authority (West Norfolk and Wisbech Area Health Authority) and the Department of Health and Social Security to court in an attempt to stop doctors from giving contraceptive advice or treatment to children under 16 without parental consent.

The case went to the High Court in 1984 where Mr Justice Woolf dismissed Mrs Gillick's claims. The Court of Appeal reversed this decision, but in 1985 it went to the House of Lords and the Law Lords ruled in favour of the original judgement delivered by Mr Justice Woolf.

MANAGEMENT

The Fraser guidelines refer to the guidelines set out by Lord Fraser in his judgement of the Gillick case in the House of Lords (1985), which apply specifically to contraceptive advice. Lord Fraser stated that a doctor could proceed to give advice and treatment:

"provided he is satisfied in the following criteria:

    1. That the girl (although under the age of 16 years of age) will understand his advice;

    2. That he cannot persuade her to inform her parents or to allow him to inform the parents that she is seeking contraceptive advice;

    3. That she is very likely to continue having sexual intercourse with or without contraceptive treatment;

    4. That unless she receives contraceptive advice or treatment her physical or mental health or both are likely to suffer;

    5. That her best interests require him to give her contraceptive advice, treatment or both without the parental consent." (Gillick v West Norfolk, 1985)

When is a child deemed competent to refuse treatment?

This is where things get a bit complicated. Although capacity to consent and to refuse treatment would appear two sides of the same coin, the courts have ruled that a refusal of treatment by a competent person under the age of 18 is not necessarily binding. In some circumstances, particularly if the young person's life is at stake, doctors may still be able to provide treatment that is in his or her best interests but legal advice should be sought.

Where a competent young person refuses treatment, the harm caused by overriding his or her choice and possibly using restraint will need to be balanced against the harm caused by failing to treat.

Parents cannot override the competent consent of a young person to treatment that you consider is in their best interests. But you can rely on parental consent when a child lacks the capacity to consent. In Scotland parents cannot authorise treatment a competent young person has refused. In England, Wales and Northern Ireland, the law on parents overriding young people's competent refusal is complex. You should seek legal advice if you think treatment is in the best interests of a competent young person who refuses.

Who has parental responsibility?

Parental responsibility is a legal concept relating to the authority to make decisions on behalf of children. Not all biological parents have parental responsibility. In relation to children born after 1 December 2003, both of a child's biological parents have parental responsibility if they are registered on a child's birth certificate. In relation to children born before this date, both of a child's parents only acquire parental responsibility if they were married at the time of the child's conception. If the parents were not married, only the mother automatically has parental responsibility, but the father may acquire it by order or agreement.

If the surgeons want to go against the parents, what is the process?

A second opinion should be provided, but it may be necessary to seek legal advice and it may be necessary to go through the courts. In the interim, only emergency treatment that is essential to preserve life or prevent serious deterioration should be provided.

What are the potential consequences of going against a parent's wishes?

Although it is in the patients best interest, going against parental wishes could severely damage the medical teams relationship with them. Ongoing communication and involvement of the parents in their child's care may help mend this relationship by explaining to the parents why the decision was made to go against them and then hopefully demonstrate the benefits of such a decision by the improvement in the medical condition of their child.

SUMMARY

Consenting a child highlights several complex issues and situations involving minors are likely to be very emotive. It is important to mention that you would inform your seniors and gain a second opinion in a timely manner as this will become vital if it escalates to challenging the parent's right to refuse consent. A child consenting for themselves is also complex, particularly when they are refusing to consent but have been deemed competent.

TOP TIPS

➕ Involve seniors and other relevant medical professionals early.

➕ Remember that the child may be able to consent for themselves - although Gillick competence and Fraser guidelines are in relation to contraception they are well known and a familiarity with them will be useful.

➕ Know the legal stance if parents continue to refuse consent but a child's life is endanger. It feels uncomfortable to say that you would go against a parent's wishes but your first priority is the safety of your patient.

MANAGEMENT

4.9 | Bullying

Scenario

You are an SHO working as part of the plastic surgery team. During your first week one of the male consultants makes a sexist remark towards a female SHO who is also apart of your team. This consultant continues to have an overtly sexist attitude towards this one particular SHO. He frequently dismisses her input on the ward round and instead openly favours the male members of the team. This is noticed by the nursing staff and on a couple of occasions he has made sexist comments in front of patients.

How would you approach this situation?

Seek Information: If you have been hearing other members of staff discuss this situation then it may be useful to ascertain how they feel about it. However, this needs to be dealt with delicately and not be seen to be digging for information or gossiping. If the SHO in question seems affected by the consultant's attitude to them then it would be reasonable to offer them support and ask if they wish to discuss any of their concerns with you informally.

Patient Safety: If a patient mentions to you that they were affected by the consultant's attitude then you should apologise for anything that made them feel uncomfortable and emphasis that that type of attitude is not something that is encouraged in the medical profession.

Initiative: Again, you need to be available to your colleague as someone to talk to. You could investigate how best to escalate the situation should your colleague wish to do so. If you feel that the situation is affecting patient care then you would be justified in escalating the situation yourself.

Escalate: If you feel that you require more senior support then it would be sensible to escalate this to your educational supervisor. In the first instance it may be an idea to keep the individuals involved anonymous and just use this opportunity to gain some advice about the situation in general. You should also encourage the SHO involved to discuss the situation with her supervisor as well for support.

Support: As above, escalating the situation to supervisor level should offer more support. You could also access support through human resources. Throughout your medical career it is also important to have a good support system outside of work. Friends and family may be able to offer impartial advice although you should ensure that you keep all people involved anonymous.

What are the key issues in this scenario?

The key issue here is lack of professionalism, in particular: bullying, harassment and victimisation.

After a ward round during which the consultant was particularly dismissive towards the SHO in question despite her trying to tell him relevant information, she confides in you that she is feeling upset and her confidence in her work is being affected. She would like to talk to someone about it but is concerned about being labelled a 'trouble-maker' and does not know the best way to deal with the situation.

Who is the best person for the SHO to talk to about this?

Your educational and clinical supervisors should be available for discussing any issues that you have with your work.

If the educational supervisor is not available where else can the SHO access advice and support?

All trainees should have an educational supervisor whom they should feel able to approach. Trainees who do not believe that this is possible or appropriate may wish to discuss the matter with the clinical director of their department. Other people in positions of responsibility who may be approached include college tutors, medical directors, or postgraduate deanery staff, such as a head of school.

Following discussion with her supervisor the SHO feels that she is justified in putting in a formal complaint. How should she go about this?

In the first instance it is advisable to contact your HR department to see if there is a harassment and bullying policy readily available. If you are uncomfortable contacting your HR department at this juncture you should contact your local BMA office to see if they have a policy for your employer or ask them to contact your HR department for this reason. If you believe that you are being subjected to bullying or harassment, you should consider keeping a diary of events, including the date/time, what happened and who was present as this will be very helpful for any action you may want to take.

What is bullying?

Bullying is where an individual or group abuses a position of power or authority over another person or persons that leaves the victim(s) feeling hurt, vulnerable, angry, or powerless.
Bullying includes but is not limited to:

- Aggression, including threats, shouting abuse and obscenities and shouting at people to get work done.
- Persistent humiliation, ridicule or criticism in front of patients, colleagues or alone.
- Malicious rumours.
- Unjustifiably changing areas of responsibility and relegating people to demeaning and inappropriate tasks.

MANAGEMENT

- Deliberately excluding the individual from discussions or decisions.
- Aggressive communication of any form, including electronic communication

What is harassment?

Harassment can take many forms and may be an isolated incident or a persistent and ongoing form of abuse. Harassment may be directed towards an individual or group of individuals and may be related to their age, sex, race, disability, religion, sexual orientation, nationality or any personal characteristic.

It may be carried out by an individual, a group of individuals or a third party (person or people who are not employees of the organisation).

'It is any behaviour, whether verbal, non-verbal, or physical, which has the purpose or effect of violating an individuals dignity or creating an intimidating, humiliating or offensive environment for that individual or group'.

What is unlawful victimisation?

This occurs where a person is treated less favourably because they have asserted their rights, perhaps through making a complaint, supporting a claimant or raising a grievance.
In some instances, it may occur as the individual is suspected to have or be considering raising a grievance. It is worth remembering that as an employee, it is within your rights to make a complaint or assist in an investigation and you are protected by law from victimisation should you do so.
Victimisation includes but is not limited to:

- Refusing reasonable requests such as unjustifiably blocking access to promotion.
- Refusing access to training or continuing profession development.
- Selecting a person for redundancy without proper justification.
- Subjecting a person to unwarranted disciplinary action.
- Subjecting a person to any other detriment.

What legislation is relevant in this case?

Harassment is held to be discrimination under the Equality Act 2010, which has harmonised the provisions for discrimination based on association or perception and indirect discrimination and protects against discrimination based on any of the following characteristics: age, disability, gender reassignment, marriage or civil partnership, pregnancy or maternity, race, religion or belief, sex and sexual orientation.

Harassment is also prohibited under the Criminal Justice and Public Order Act 1994, which makes intentional harassment a criminal offence. The Protection from Harassment Act 1997 makes it a criminal offence to pursue a course of conduct, which amounts to harassment of a person, or which causes a person to fear that violence will be used against them.

MANAGEMENT

What is the formal complaints process?

Informal action is normally a very effective method of dealing with cases of bullying and harassment, but if you feel that you cannot find a resolution via this channel or you have been unsuccessful previously you may feel the need to take formal action. You should seek advice from your local BMA office before taking formal action. You may also wish to take additional advice or counselling at this stage. The following sets out a model process:

- If the incident is isolated it is important to create a written report of the event with as much detail as possible and name any witnesses, if appropriate.
- Make a verbal or written complaint sent in confidence to the HR department. You may wish to get assistance or representation from the BMA, your line manager, if appropriate, the HR manager or a staff representative.

An investigative process should begin, with the involvement of the HR team if required. Where a case to answer has been found, formal disciplinary procedure against the harasser or bully should be commenced, depending on the case and employer.

Where a possible criminal offence has been disclosed, the police should be informed of the allegation.

SUMMARY

Being a victim of bullying or harassment can be extremely damaging emotional, psychologically and potentially professionally. It is important that you seek support and advice early on and escalate it as required. If you do feel that the situation can not be resolved informally then you should know who in your trust to contact to start a formal process. In the event of a formal complaint, having examples of when you have been bullied, harassed or victimised may help with the process.

TOP TIPS

 Knowing definitions of the various types of unprofessional behaviour should help you get the nature of a scenario clear in your head.

 Do not underestimate the role of your supervisors; they should ideally be the first port of call when looking for advice with difficulties at work.

MANAGEMENT

4.10 Difficult Colleague

Scenario

You are a CT1 in plastic surgery. You notice on the new rota sent out, that the staff grade SHO in charge of the rota has given himself 10 extra free days for the next 6-month rotation on top of his given annual leave and study leave meaning that the rest of the SHOs are going to have to cover his ward work.

What would you do?

Seek Information: You need to firstly ensure that you have correctly identified that the SHO has taken more days than allowed, and whether he has been entitled to those zero days in advance.

Patient Safety: Patient safety is at risk with a reduction in doctor cover caused by absence due to the increased workload on the rest of the team.

Initiative: It would be important to act quickly before the effects of the rota are felt and to raise the issue with the SHO in question and fellow team members

Escalate: If necessary you would need to escalate the situation to the consultant/line manager who gives authorisation for leave.

Support: It would be important to support the SHO to ensure that the rota is correct and accurate, especially as this situation may be a genuine mistake.

The SHO responds by stating that he needs the extra time off to write up his dissertation for his PhD.

What are the key issues?

The main issue is firstly probity, as the doctor has unfairly given himself more that the allocated time off for a personal reason. Secondly there is an issue of patient safety as other doctors are going to have to cover more patients allowing scope for mistakes to be made. Thirdly, it is unfair on the rest of the SHOs as they will be overworked and are not given the same amount of time off.

What would you do?

Now that you have a reason for the situation, it is important for discussion to be had with the SHO in question about the main issues in order to bring it to his attention. It would also be vital to discuss these issues with the other SHOs involved to seek their opinion and support. If they were not amenable to making changes, you would need to flag this issue to an appropriate senior colleague or manager.

What strategies can you use to help support this colleague during this time?

It is important that you support your colleagues through difficult periods, particularly if it is short term, however this should not be at the detriment of patient safety. It would be important to suggest that the SHO use their annual leave and study leave allocation to ensure that the work is done, and help him improve his time management. You could offer to help cover some of his duties during the working week along with the rest of the team for a short period of time to give him some extra time e.g. holding his bleep for an hour in the day.

The consultant in charge of approving leave allocation is also the PhD supervisor for the SHO in question and has approved the extra leave for the SHO.

What issues does this raise?

There is a possibility that a conflict of interest is present, as the consultant may be very keen for the SHO to complete the dissertation. However despite this, the consultant should recognise the probity and patient safety issues raised. Approving the leave, does not automatically mean the consultant is aware of the implications. You may need to discuss the issues raised from the SHO's absence with the consultant before concluding that he knows about the situation.

Who else could you escalate this issue to?

It is always important to escalate issues that affect you in the workplace to your direct line manager, either the consultant you work for, or your clinical supervisor before involving any other senior management. If this is unsuccessful, it would be important to talk to a departmental or service manager in order to raise the issue to.

What is probity?

Probity means being honest and trustworthy, acting with integrity. The GMC highlights this as an important characteristic for all doctors to have in order to make sure that their behaviour justifies the trust the public hold in us.

Why is probity in medicine important?

Probity is important as it allows us to have a strong moral standing for which the public can base their trust in the medical profession. It is also important for us to be honest with not only patients, but with each other as professionals as we often work as part of a team and need to maintain relationships within the team environment.

SUMMARY

Being a rota coordinator is a difficult job in order to balance expectations and mange a team, however the power and responsibility that comes with it should never be abused. Probity is a principle which not only applies to our patients but also to our colleagues. We should aim to be honest with our colleagues in order to maintain relationships, build trust and support each other for the benefit of our patients.

MANAGEMENT

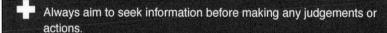

TOP TIPS

➕ Always aim to seek information before making any judgements or actions.

➕ If a colleague has an issue or problem, always think about methods to support that colleague prior to full escalation.

4.11   Difficult Patient

Scenario

You are a CT1 in urology. There is a commotion in the reception of the outpatient clinic and one of the nurses comes into your clinic room to ask if you can speak to an angry patient outside. She reports that the patient only wants to be seen by a 'white' doctor. There are currently no other doctors except the registrar and consultant who are neither white nor from the UK.

How would you approach this situation?

Seek Information: It would be important not to rush into the situation without adequate information. What is the underlying problem? Is the patient intoxicated? Have they been waiting or have another issue?

Patient Safety: You want to minimise disruption and anxiety to patients waiting and ensure that his anger is not turned to anyone in the waiting area.

Initiative: Is there anything that you can do immediately to calm things. Can he be persuaded to go to a side room? Is he likely to be amenable to calm discussion?

Escalate: Ensure that a senior member of staff is informed if the issue cannot be resolved immediately. In extreme cases where he is causing disruption to the hospital environment asking him to leave or calling for security may be appropriate.

Support: It is also important to be supportive to the patient and remind the patient that the team are here to help and are all sufficiently qualified to see him.

What steps would you take to prevent confrontation?

In order to avoid confrontation in this situation you will need to make the patient involved feel that their concerns are being heard. It would be important to take the patient to a quieter area, where you can discuss the situation further without interference. You will need to maintain a neutral stance throughout any discussion and avoid any judgemental language or behaviour towards the patient. However it would be important to remind the patient that discriminatory behaviour is not tolerated. You will then attempt to come up with a mutually acceptable

MANAGEMENT

solution.

Is the patient allowed to request who he sees in clinic?

The patient is within his rights to request to see a particular doctor if they have a reasonable reason, particularly in specialities where their problems may be more sensitive, however this does not include discrimination on the basis of race, and any racism should not be tolerated. Attempts should be made to reassure the patient, and if there is a sensible reason, alternative arrangements made.

The patient becomes verbally abusive towards you and the nurse.

What are the potential issues raised by this patient's behaviour?

The patient being verbally abusive indicates that there has been an escalation in the situation and the patient could now be a danger to others as well as himself if his behaviour continues. It would be important to recognise this, and ensure that the situation is dealt with swiftly and precautions taken, such as ensuring the discussion happens away from other patients.

How would you handle this situation?

Abuse of any sort is not tolerated towards staff, however it is important to recognise that the patient may be distressed by the current handling of the situation. You need to stay calm, letting the patient know that you are there to help and that you do not want any confrontation. Calling for assistance if you felt that you could no longer manage the situation is vital. Being antagonist or just walking away from the situation would not be ideal.

Who would you call to assist you in dealing with this patient?

Firstly you could call on assistance from any family and/or friends who came with the patient to help calm the patient down. Secondly the registrar or consultant in clinic could be helpful in providing assistance in allaying this patient's fear. Thirdly security may need to be called in order to help control the situation if there is any further escalation.

The patient attempts to hit you. What would you do?

The most important thing would be to protect yourself as best as possible. Retaliation is unacceptable, however force could be used in self-defence to protect yourself. Ideally you should leave the area to avoid further assault and contacting security in order to help remove the patient as soon as possible. You should not tolerate any form of physical abuse. It would be important to inform the police of any physical assault and to report the incident via formal hospital incident reporting protocols.

Can you use physical force to restrain patients in a hospital setting?

Physical intervention should be used as a last resort, and as part of a broader strategy to manage behaviour of those who pose a risk to themselves or to oth-

MANAGEMENT

ers. Within reason physical force may be used to restrain or move patients in a hospital environment. However this should be carried out by trained members of staff if they are a danger to others around them. Ideally the police should be called in any instance where physical abuse is an issue to offer assistance. If the patient had been acutely unwell on ward.

What steps could be taken to protect the patient and those around them?

Personal care plans can be a useful way of managing patients with challenging behaviour on wards, especially if they do not have capacity at the time. This can include managing the patient in a side room or with one to one nursing care. Sedation is a last resort and should only be used if the patient is at risk of harming themselves and all steps have been taken to prevent this from happening. You could refer to your local guidelines on managing aggressive patients.

What could be the cause(s) of his behaviour?

Aggression from an acutely unwell patient may be due to a number of medical, psychiatric or emotional reasons. In patients who are acutely unwell on the ward, it is important to think about their baseline function and its impact e.g. dementia. You should consider whether their condition may be causing a delirium or if their pain is causing distress. Excluding a medical cause is vital in managing the patient appropriately.

SUMMARY

Discrimination of any sort should not be tolerated within the NHS, towards staff or patients. The Equality Act 2010 outlines what constitutes discrimination and and what is therefore unacceptable. Dealing with conflict, particularly when it involves patients is a key skill to master as a doctor at all levels. Respect, empathy and good communication are key to dealing with such situations even when a patient is in the wrong.

TOP TIPS

➕ Physical abuse should never be tolerated. You have an obligation to protect yourself, staff and patients from inappropriate aggression, so consider the safest options.

➕ Physical intervention should only be used as a last resort. Consider other forms of support for relevant patients prior to restraint.

MANAGEMENT

4.12 | Limited Resources

> **Scenario**
>
> You are a CT2 in general surgery. You have been called to a trauma call in the emergency department resus area at a trauma unit. A young man has had a crush injury following an RTA and has a possible flail chest and requires admission. Unfortunately there are currently bed shortages in the hospital and ambulances are currently being diverted away from the hospital.

How would you approach this patient?

Seek Information: This patient needs to be managed according to ATLS protocol, ensuring that C-spine protection and airway support is in place as required and that he is receiving supplementary oxygen. You need to clarify what the bed situation is.

Patient Safety: You need to ascertain his clinical priority and stability. Is he stable? Would he survive transfer?

Initiative: You need to assess the patient's breathing and the patient's circulation, disability and exposure and assess stability. Speak to the bed managers, the A&E doctors and consultant and your consultant.

Escalate: You are not alone and this shouldn't be down to you to make a decision. Involve appropriate seniors.

Support: Ensure that you keep both the patient and relatives informed and reflect on the incident and learn from it for the future.

What are the main issues regarding this situation?

Firstly the patient's clinical condition is the main issue to consider in this situation and it would be important to fully assess and manage the patient appropriately and ensure that he is haemodynamically stable. Secondly, the bed shortage poses a possible situation in terms of admitting the patient once they have been managed in the emergency department as he will need to be monitored and will need regular analgesia.

What are your primary concerns regarding this patient's condition?

Due to his suspected pathology, his breathing will be of primary concern, and will need supplementary oxygen and possible respiratory support. Once his breathing is managed, it would be important to ensure his circulation is adequate and that there is no blood loss from elsewhere. A thorough secondary survey will also be vital to avoid missing any other injuries.

Who needs to be involved in decision making for the admission of this patient?

The decision to admit the patient resides with the on-call surgical registrar who

MANAGEMENT

has the clinical responsibility for admission. Discussion will need to be had with the bed manager and the clinical site manager regarding the appropriate ward for admission. The emergency department nurse in charge will also need to be informed of progress to organise the admission of the patient.

There are no beds at all in the hospital and the patient will require admission. Who could you escalate this situation to?

It would be advisable to ensure that the on-call registrar is aware and has possibly reviewed the patient to ensure senior involvement. It would be important that the consultant on call is also aware of the situation. The clinical site manager and bed manager will need to be informed and discussions regarding possible solutions should be had with them.

What measures could you suggest to help allow this patient to be admitted?

It should be primarily the responsibility of the bed manager to find a bed for the patient on a suitable ward, however it may be possible to help by reviewing patients under your team's care who may possibly go home, thereby allowing a surgical bed to be available.

What is "bed-blocking" and how is it affecting the NHS?

"Bed-blocking" is the term used to describe the loss of acute hospital bed space due to patients awaiting social care input in their discharge. This is usually due to delayed discharging and relates particularly to the elderly population and those with special needs. This results in a backlog in emergency admissions, preventing patients from being seen and admitted from the emergency department within recommended targets. Inevitably, this has an effect on emergency patient care. It has been suggested that greater emphasis and spending on social care, may improve this phenomena and ease pressure on emergency departments.

You are asked to refer this patient to the nearby major trauma centre. What information do you need to give as part of this referral?

In order to give the best description of the clinical picture an SBAR (situation, background, assessment, recommendation) structured handover can be used to give information to the receiving doctor. This highlights the main problems with his clinical condition, including most recent observations and oxygen requirements, any interventions done or currently active including any lines or devices inserted.

What important information do you need to gain when making the referral?

Firstly you need to clarify who you are referring to and who is accepting the referral, including title, full name and speciality. You need to ensure that you come to agreement about the referral status and clarify where the patient needs to be sent to when transferred e.g. ward, A&E. Finally you will need to establish if there are any further actions which need to be completed prior to transfer, e.g. interventions, imaging etc.

The patient is now haemodynamically unstable and is unable to maintain oxygenation. What would you do?

You would need to re-assess the patient as per ATLS guidelines, assessing his airway, breathing and circulation. You may need to repeat investigations such as a chest xray and it would be important to contact the anaesthetic team to obtain help for his airway and also intensive care as the patient may require ventilator support. If the patient does need to be intubated, this should not affect any transfer once he has been stabilised and his cardiovascular parameters are controlled.

SUMMARY

In today's modern NHS, bed shortages and limited resources are becoming more commonplace. It is important to ensure that you do as much as possible to ensure the best care for the patient and all should be done to accommodate the patient with minimal disruption in their emergency care. According to ATLS guidelines, primary survey should still be completed prior to transfer to stabilise the patient.

TOP TIPS

➕ Think about local solutions to resourcing problems in order to accommodate admission of patients.

➕ Remember to ensure that the patient is properly assessed and managed appropriately, even if there is the possibility of transfer.

➕ When discussing patients or handing over information, SBAR is a vital tool in ensuring you cover the essential points.

MANAGEMENT

4.13 | Negotiating

> ## Scenario
>
> You are a CT2 SHO in general surgery. You have admitted a 65-year-old woman who is acutely unwell and has a peritonitic abdomen. She requires an emergency laparotomy and needs to be done urgently in the NCEPOD emergency theatre. At the same time, the gynaecology team have a 24-year-old female who has a possible ectopic pregnancy who they also want to take to theatre.

How would you prepare this patient for theatre?

You will firstly need to resuscitate the patient prior to theatre and ensure that all relevant blood results are available and that the patient is fasted. It would be important to ensure that she has an up-to-date group and save and that the patient is cross-matched at least 2 units of blood as she will be having a major operation. She will need to be consented and discussion with her and relevant family members will also be needed.

You will have to ensure that the theatre coordinator and staff are aware of the patient and that the anaesthetist on call is available for the case. Discussion with the gynaecology team will then need to take place regarding which patient will be operated on first.

What information would you want to help decide which patient should be prioritised?

You would want to know the haemodynamic status of both patients in order to decide who is more critically unwell at the time as well as their response to any conservative or medical interventions. Any relevant blood results would also be useful, as this could give further indication of urgency, e.g. blood loss (haemoglobin), ischaemia (lactate).

Any outstanding issues which may cause a delay, e.g. adjusting pacemaker settings, may allow the other speciality to go first.

Length of procedure may also help decide, e.g. a laparotomy for faecal peritonitis will take considerably longer than a laparoscopic salpingectomy. Imaging may be useful if available to help decide on clinical status.

Who would you need to involve to make a decision about who goes to theatre first?

It would be important to hold discussions with the gynaecology team, the anaesthetist on call and the theatre coordinator in order to decide on what the best course of action is. It is necessary to escalate the issue to the relevant consultants of the involved teams to ensure that they are aware in case the situation takes a turn for the worse.

MANAGEMENT

What options could be considered to resolve this issue?

Another theatre could be opened to enable both procedures to take place and avoid delay in both patient's care. It would be important to discuss this option with the theatre coordinator and anaesthetics team, as this may be possible if there are enough staff members present. If there are not enough staff members, it may be important to escalate this issue to the clinical site manager who may be able to provide further staff from another environment at short notice to cover, enabling both surgeries to occur.

What possible outcomes are available?

The best outcome for both patients would be both to be operated on at the same time in two different theatres with the right amount of staff present. However if this is not possible, the least compromised patient could be optimised carefully in preparation for theatre while the most urgent case is done, with as minimal disruption as possible. If available and safe, further imaging could be obtained such as a CT scan to gain further information about each patient.

Both patients are currently haemodynamically unstable and require urgent operations. The gynaecology registrar is adamant that their patient is more unwell.

Who would you escalate this issue to?

It would be vital at this stage to involve the consultants from all 3 specialities, including general surgery, gynaecology and anaesthetics as well as the clinical site manager. The final decision regarding which patient goes to theatre first would rest with them as the most senior clinicians.

What is NCEPOD? What impact has it had on surgical practice?

NCEPOD stands for the national confidential enquiry into peri-operative deaths. Its introduction has led to improvements in surgical safety, particularly emergency surgery. Following its investigation, it suggests that operations should not take place out of hours if they can be avoided.

What are the CEPOD categories? What are they used for?

Each emergency case must be assessed for urgency and hence appropriately positioned on the operating list. The 4 main CEPOD categories characterise an operation's urgency. These are immediate, urgent, expedited and elective. This allows clinicians and managers who are responsible for allocating theatre time to prioritise accordingly.

You arrive with the surgical registrar to consent the patient however the 65-year-old woman appears to be delirious and does not know where she is and so therefore no longer has capacity to consent. What options are available?

All attempts must be made to establish whether the patient has capacity, and in the emergency setting, it would be appropriate to discuss with the patient's

MANAGEMENT

relatives and relevant friends to ascertain what the patient would have wanted if they were competent. Other sources such as advance directives may be useful in determining wishes. If unable to determine wishes through these means, the patient must then be treated as being unable to give consent.

Are doctors allowed to carry out operations without patients' consent?

The doctor can treat the patient on the basis that the treatment administered is limited to what is immediately necessary to save the patient's life or prevent serious deterioration of their condition.

SUMMARY

Negotiating with other specialties for various reasons, including use of resources and referrals is a vital part of the daily job. It is important to always put the patient's interests first. Finding a solution requires discussion and assistance from all parties involved and should take place in order to minimise harm.

TOP TIPS

➕ Always seek to involve theatre coordinators, anaesthetists and other surgeons in discussion regarding taking patients to theatre.

➕ The urgency of an operative procedure can be graded according to CEPOD criteria, however it is important to note that the clinical picture is important in making the final decision.

➕ In patients who are unable to give consent, emergency procedures should still be carried out if in patient's best interest.

MANAGEMENT

How would you approach this scenario?

4.14 | Wrong Site Surgery

Scenario

You are the general surgery SHO on-call when a patient you had incorrectly marked had the wrong lump removed. The patient is still unaware of the mistake. On reflection you remember that you were very busy on the day the mistake was made. The patient is still an inpatient in the hospital. The relatives of the patient have requested to speak with you.

Seek Information: In this challenging scenario it is important that the patient receives accurate and truthful information from healthcare professionals responsible for their care.

Patient Safety: The first steps in this case will include recognising that this incident has had a direct impact on patient in terms of harm.

Initiative: It is important to notify the patient that an adverse event has occurred at the earliest opportunity. In order to facilitate this process you need to ensure that your registrar and consultant are aware of the event.

Escalate: The next step would be to notify the patient. Ideally this should be conducted in an open discussion with the most senior member of the team being present.

Support: The patient and their family should be provided with a step-by-step explanation of the events that had taken place. An apology should be offered to the patient and further support for the patient should be explored and discussed.

What are the key issues?

Honesty and integrity
Duty of candour
Communication with patients and relatives
Incident reporting

The patient has expressed that they are concerned by the events that have occurred and wish to continue treatment with another team. How would you proceed?

The patient has the right to request that another physician take over their care. You should endeavour to ensure that this is made possible. You should reassure the patient that they will receive all usual treatment and will continue to be treated with dignity, respect and compassion.

Following on from your discussions, the patient has informed you that he wishes to make a formal complaint. What do you know about the complaints process in the hospital?

In the event where a patient wishes to make a complaint the patient advice and liaison service (PALS) offers confidential advice, support and information on health related matters. They provide a point of contact for patients, their families

MANAGEMENT

and their carers.

What steps can be taken as a junior doctor to report incidents that have had an adverse effect on patient safety?

As a junior doctor there are many avenues that are available for incident reporting. One such avenue is the local NHS trusts incident report form. These are usually accessible on the trust intranet or on the wards in paper form. In addition to this addressing the situation with the clinical lead for the department and your clinical supervisor will help to ensure that the situation is appropriately escalated. From an educational perspective it is always important to try and implement changes that will prevent adverse events from occurring again. Audits and quality improvement projects are an avenue of reporting changes and implementing positive change. Mortality and morbidity meetings are held regularly in surgical departments this is also an avenue for incident reporting.

What do you understand about the duty of candour?

The duty of candour is a legal duty on hospital, community and mental health trusts to inform and apologise to patients if there have been mistakes in their care that have led to harm.

What surgical checklists are you aware of that can be used to prevent wrong site surgery?

The WHO surgical checklist

What are the steps of WHO surgical checklist?

There are 3 main components of the WHO surgical checklist. The sections relate to before the induction of anaesthesia, before skin incision and before the patient leaves the room. Before the induction of anaesthesia, the identity of the patient is confirmed and the consent form, site of operation and operative procedure are checked. During this stage the operative site is marked. The amount of expected blood loss is discussed and the anaesthetic safety check is completed.

Before the first skin incision the entire team are required to pause whilst one member of the team will read the "time out". Each member within the operating theatre will introduce themselves and their role. The name of the patient and the procedure that is taking place are discussed along with any anticipated critical events or special equipment required. At this point antibiotic prophylaxis, hair removal and diabetic control are all considered on an individual case basis.

After the operation, before the patient leaves theatre a further check is conducted. This is usually conducted by the scrub nurse. The instruments, swabs and needle counts are checked and numbered. Any faulty equipment is noted and intraoperative specimens are appropriately labelled and sent to the necessary departments. Any key concerns for recovery are also discussed.

Outside of the surgical checklist how would you confirm the site of an operation?

This is focusing on the importance of reviewing the patient before an operation. A detailed history and examination with a review of the clinic notes is always advised before performing or assisting in any surgical procedure and will reduce the risk of wrong site surgery.

SUMMARY

Following the Francis report into the events at mid Staffordshire NHS trust there has been a call within the NHS for the establishment of a statutory duty of candour. It is important to be truthful with patients about the care they are being provided. Safety checklists help to reduce adverse events and are important aspect of patient safety.

TOP TIPS

➕ A good awareness of duty of candour will score well in this scenario.

➕ Be aware of the clinical incident reporting system.

➕ A common pitfall here would be to avoid disclosing the information, this would be a breach of the duty of candour and would not stand well at interview.

MANAGEMENT

4.15 Absent Colleague

Scenario

You are the general surgical SHO on-call for the day. Following an intense on-call shift you are due to handover when you notice that the night SHO has not arrived. You have a list of patients in A&E who are waiting to be seen and a particularly unwell patient on the ward. You have not received any information from the night SHO.

How would you approach this scenario?

Seek Information: This is a challenging situation for any trainee. A thorough assessment of the situation will help you to clarify what actions you need to take.
Patient Safety: Clearly someone needs to cover the wards and shift in order to maintain patient safety and the person covering the shift should not be tired or at risk of making mistakes.
Initiative: Establishing communication between yourself and your colleague will help to determine an expected time of arrival or if there is a problem. Do you know any of his/her housemates if he/she is not answering their phone? You can demonstrate further initiative by prioritising which patients need to be seen most urgently to ensure an effective handover.
Escalate: Alternatively one can contact medical staffing or the site manager to determine whether there has been any contact from your colleague regarding their attendance to hospital. Let your registrar and consultant know and see if you can come up with a plan.
Support: Find out the reason behind the colleagues unreported absence. Is there an underlying problem that needs dealing with?

What are the key issues?

Patient safety
Appropriate escalation of staffing issues
Support for your colleague

You have been unable to contact your colleague and you are now 45 minutes into the night shift. How would you proceed?

Once you have assessed the situation, you must make sure that patient safety is at the forefront of any decision you choose to take. An awareness of your own limitations will help to protect your patients. If you feel that you are too tired to continue the shift as the night SHO, then the night team should be informed as you are under no obligation to do so. You can demonstrate further initiative by prioritising which patients need to be seen most urgently to ensure an effective handover. You can escalate your concerns to the Consultant on-call. Most hospitals within the NHS employ a step down policy where the Consultant will perform the duties of the registrar, whilst the registrar performs the duty of the SHO.

Who can you contact in the hospital to raise concerns about staffing issues?

Clinical lead for the department would be an appropriate step in raising concerns with regards to staffing issues. The medical staffing department are also available for staffing issues that may arise. A trainee may also find it beneficial to contact their line manager. You may find it useful to inform your clinical supervisor as staffing issues may have a detrimental effect on patient safety and your ability to perform your duties.

You notice that your colleague has regularly been 2 hours late for his last 3 night on-call shifts. How would you proceed?

This question is really focussing on your ability to support your colleague and escalate any problems appropriately. In this case it is necessary to identify with your colleague if there are any ongoing issues or difficulties that they may be facing. It is important to do this in a non-confrontational manner within a relaxed environment. Explain to your colleague that you have noticed a recent tendency to arrive late and that you are duly concerned. Discuss the effect that this may have on patient safety and ensure that any support that is required is promptly sought. There may be a number of reasons for this recent development and it is important to establish that any support can be provided promptly.

Your colleague informs you that he has been having difficulties with childcare in the evenings and has been late every night as a result. What support is available within the hospital for a trainee who is struggling with personal problems?

Occupational health would be an appropriate avenue for a trainee with any concerns with regards to their health. Clinical and educational supervisors are available to support trainees in any capacity. If a trainee is still having difficulties despite exploring these avenues then a trainee may be able to contact the training programme director for further support.

What organisations are available to provide advice for junior doctors in difficulties?

Organisations such as the BMA, the GMC or any medical defence organisation are available to support junior doctors in difficulties. They are able to provide telephone consultations or face-to-face meetings for trainees. There are also organisations outside of medicine that help with personal problems that a trainee may decide to explore.

SUMMARY

This is a challenging scenario and is testing your ability to maintain patient safety whilst supporting your colleagues. A good working knowledge of how to escalate staffing issues in the hospital will score well in this scenario. A trainee should be aware of how to raise concerns about their colleagues and offer suggestions for avenues of support.

MANAGEMENT

TOP TIPS

➕ In this scenario the SPIES technique will help you to structure your answer.

➕ Knowledge of support services will be useful for this scenario and life in general.

➕ Always remember to support your colleagues who are in difficulty.

Printed in Great Britain
by Amazon